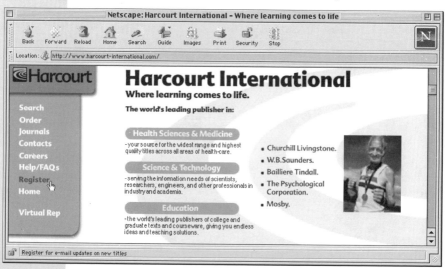

Women's Health: A Handbook for Nurses

Catriona Sutherland RGN ENB A08, A51, 998
Practice Nurse and Nurse Specialist in Women's Health,
Paxton Green Group Practice, London;
Member of Steering Group of RCN Sexual Health Forum,
London, UK

Edited by

Sue Hinchliff BA MSc RGN RN
Head of Accreditation,
Royal College of Nursing of the United Kingdom,
London, UK

Rosemary Rogers BA RGN
Publishing Director, Emap
Healthcare Open Learning,
London, UK

Foreword by

Jacqui Fletcher BSc(Hons) PGCert RGN
Senior Lecturer Tissue Viability, Department
of Health Registration Nursing,
University of Hertfordshire,
Hatfield, UK

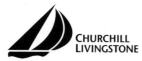

CHURCHILL
LIVINGSTONE

EDINBURGH LONDON NEW YORK PHILADELPHIA ST LOUIS SYDNEY TORONTO 2001

CHURCHILL LIVINGSTONE
An imprint of Harcourt Publishers Limited

First published 2001

ISBN 0 443 06176 9

British Library Cataloguing in Publication Data
A catalogue record for this book is available from the British Library

Library of Congress Cataloging in Publication Data
A catalog record for this book is available from the Library of Congress

Note
Medical knowledge is constantly changing. As new information becomes available, changes in treatment, procedures, equipment and the use of drugs become necessary. The author and the publishers have taken care to ensure that the information given in this text is accurate and up to date. However, readers are strongly advised to confirm that the information, especially with regard to drug usage, complies with the latest legislation and standards of practice.

The
publisher's
policy is to use
**paper manufactured
from sustainable forests**

Printed in China

Contents

Foreword

Within the current climate of the National Health Service considerable emphasis is placed on the use of evidence based practice (Mead 2000). It is widely accepted, however, that implementation of evidence based practice is a lengthy and complicated process (Wye & McClenahan 2000) and the outcomes of this implementation are rarely evaluated fully. A systematic review of clinical guidelines as a means of implementing evidence based practice over the last twenty-five years was able to identify only eighteen studies that met the inclusion criteria, only two of which studies were relevant to women's health needs (Thomas et al 1999).

Cullum et al (1997) clearly identified the role nurses have in the identification of patients' actual and potential health needs and in making a difference to the outcomes of patients' care; however, they also highlighted the many difficulties nurses experience in implementing research findings in their day-to-day practice, suggesting that nurses have difficulty in accessing and appraising published data. This is compounded by the belief of many that evidence based care is the province of the medical practitioner, with less attention being focused on multidisciplinary or more holistic approaches to care; indeed, some authors suggest that the emphasis on evidence based medicine (as opposed to evidence based practice) may have a deleterious effect on the development of nursing and health care (French 1999). When considering the development of evidence based nursing, Closs and Cheater (1999) caution that there are many complexities to be considered and that, given the relatively small amounts of good-quality evidence available, it is currently unrealistic to assume that all aspects of nursing practice should be evidence based.

In view of the amount of support from the current government for evaluating both the quality of the care delivered and the outcomes of that care, this is an ideal time for healthcare practitioners to address women's needs and identify areas where inequalities and inequity exist. These are the areas where good-quality multidisciplinary research and clinical guidelines based on the outcomes of that research are desperately required. Although clinical guidelines which aim to standardize best practice are becoming more widely used in the area of women's health, with, for instance, a range of national guidelines on cervical screening having been in existence since 1994 (see 'Who is at increased risk of cervical cancer?', p. 38), it is imperative that this level of interest be maintained across all women's issues and the comments made in relation to the psychosocial and political aspects of women's health need to be awarded due attention when considering why these areas have been given such low priority to date.

This timely publication addresses both biological and gender-specific issues, highlighting the inequalities in health between men and women and also between women of different socioeconomic groups. The use of key issue boxes encourages the reader to focus on specific factors and questions the reader's knowledge base and current practice. By fostering this critical approach to care delivery, the author has produced a resource that will encourage an evidence based approach to care long after some of the techniques discussed have become out of date. It will set a pattern of working that will serve the reader for many years to come.

Jacqui Fletcher

REFERENCES

Closs SJ, Cheater FM 1999 Evidence for nursing practice: a clarification of the issues. Journal of Advanced Nursing 30(1): 10–17

Cullum N, DiCenso A, Ciliska D 1997 Evidence-based nursing: an introduction. Nursing Standard 11(28): 32–33

French P 1999 The development of evidence based nursing. Journal of Advanced Nursing 29(1): 72–78

Mead P (2000) Clinical guidelines: promoting clinical effectiveness or a professional minefield? Journal of Advanced Nursing 31(1): 100–116

Thomas LH, McColl E, Callum N, Rousseau N, Soutter J 1999 Clinical guidelines in nursing, midwifery and the therapies: a systematic review. Journal of Advanced Nursing 30(1): 40–50

Wye L, McClenahan J 2000 Getting better with evidence. Experiences of putting evidence into practice. King's Fund Publishing, London

Preface

WHAT IS WOMEN'S HEALTH?

Although we talk about women as if they were a unified group, we must always remember that women are not a single homogeneous group, as they have varied experiences, interests, needs and desires (Doyal 1998).

However, issues in women's health may be broadly grouped into four categories:

- conditions and experiences which are exclusive to women, but which are not diseases, such as pregnancy, childbirth, breastfeeding and the menopause
- disorders which are directly related to the female anatomy, such as gynaecological cancers and breast disease
- conditions which affect both sexes but which are a significant health issue for women, such as coronary heart disease, lung cancer and breast cancer
- issues which arise from women's lifestyles and experience in society, which may include mental health, sexual health and contraception (Cook 1998).

WHY IS WOMEN'S HEALTH AN ISSUE?

Everyone's health is an issue and of equal importance, but there is a body of opinion that asserts that women are treated differently and unfairly within the healthcare system. The following examples are made (Doyal 1998):

- women's own experiences are often devalued in comparison with 'expert' medical knowledge
- women may be denied the opportunity to participate fully in treatment decisions, both medical and surgical
- the reduction in family planning services has a major effect on women

- women have to negotiate with, and endure, the personal judgements of others when seeking to use fertility control
- deaths from breast cancer are unnecessarily high, owing to a lack of consistency in the standards of specialist treatment and in women's access to such treatment
- women are denied the same opportunities as men for research, investigation and treatment of coronary heart disease.

NURSING ISSUES IN WOMEN'S HEALTH

The great majority of nurses are women; therefore, we are in the privileged position of caring for someone who could be our mother, grandmother, sister, daughter, flatmate, partner or friend. Much of nursing may be about **doing** caring tasks and activities, but all of nursing is about **communication**.

Communication is a two-way process. The nurse enables the patient to communicate information about herself, her health, relationships, lifestyle, fears and needs (her psychological, cultural and psychosocial environment, as it pertains to her health issues). In return, the nurse empowers the patient by openly sharing information and facts that are known about her health care and the decisions involved in it (Firth & Watanabe 1996).

The information we share with our patients must be:

- current
- appropriate
- accessible, in terms of language
- accurate
- what the patient wants, whether or not we like it or approve of it.

One of our most important roles can be in acting as our patient's advocate. We must respect our patient's views and beliefs, which may be at odds with our own and we must not impose our views and beliefs on our patients. If we do not know something we must say so, but know where to obtain the information.

Disapproval can take many forms:

- making the patient defend or justify her behaviour
- withholding information

- patronizing
- making personal comments
- being very impersonal or even ignoring the patient
- sending non-verbal clues (by posture, gestures, facial expression, speech and tone)
- not showing respect or preserving her dignity.

USING THIS BOOK

This book is intended as a first point of reference in the process of finding out more about issues in women's health. Each section in each chapter stands alone, although it may be linked to other sections and other chapters. The references, further reading and resources are included at the end of each section.

Drugs

The British National Formulary (BNF) is an under-utilized resource, is revised twice-yearly and provides excellent guidance on prescribing. The BNF is produced by the British Medical Association and the Royal Pharmaceutical Society of Great Britain.

Drugs in Nursing Practice, 5th edn (Henney CR, Dow RJ and MacConnachie AM 1995, Churchill Livingstone, Edinburgh) identifies the contribution that nurses can make in achieving the most effective and safe use of drugs for their patients.

Nursing women

The technology, techniques and therapy may change when caring for women, but the principles of nursing care remain the same (for example, the need to maintain dignity, privacy and hygiene, and to communicate clearly and appropriately).

These two texts have nursing care plans that can be adapted to accommodate all areas of women's health:

- Edge V, Miller M (eds) 1994 Mosby's Clinical Nursing Series: Women's health care. Mosby, St Louis
- Gould D 1990 Nursing care of women. Prentice Hall, New York.

Sexuality

This is an area often denied or ignored in nursing care. I have included lesbianism in the chapter on Sensitive Issues, not because I believe that lesbianism is a sensitive issue (i.e. one requiring something out of the ordinary), but to raise awareness of the ordinary day-to-day needs of lesbian women. Homophobia and heterosexism discourage lesbians from seeking and receiving appropriate health care (Wilton 1998).

London 2001   Catriona Sutherland

REFERENCES

Cook R 1998 Promoting women's health. Primary Health Care 8 (2): 31–38
Doyal L 1998 Introduction: women and health services. In: Doyal L (ed) Women and health services. Open University Press, Buckingham
Firth PA, Watanabe SJ (eds) 1996 Instant nursing assessment: women's health. Delmar Publishers, Albany
Wilton T 1998 Gender, sexuality and healthcare: improving services. In: Doyal L (ed) Women and health services. Open University Press, Buckingham

Acknowledgements

I am most grateful to my professional colleagues for their encouragement and support, particularly Suzanne Everett.

I must also thank Norman Sutherland, whose support, patience and attention to detail have been invaluable: he now knows more about women's health than most men.

1

Psychosocial and political aspects of women's health

GENDER, STATUS AND HEALTH

It is necessary to distinguish between biological (or sexual) differences between men's and women's health and social (or gender) differences. Both are important in understanding health and illness (Doyal 1998).

There are inequalities in health between both men and women, and between women of different socio-economic status.

POVERTY (Whitehead 1992)

- Living conditions, working conditions and unemployment all have a detrimental effect on health.
- Large differences in deprivation exist between different areas of the country, as well as within much smaller administrative areas.
- Social isolation and poor social support are linked to poor mental and physical health.
- Quality of care can appear to favour higher occupational classes.
- There is lower uptake of preventive services by lower social groups.

- 'Deprived' patients may have considerably more hospital admissions, casualty attendances and mental illness.
- Socio-economic differentials in mortality in women persist at each life-cycle stage.
- Women in part-time non-manual jobs appear to have the lowest mortality in each life-cycle stage.
- Full-time work may be detrimental to women's health because of the added stress of trying to accommodate the multiple roles of housewife, mother and employee.
- People who are disadvantaged may be offered poorer quality and less effective investigation, treatment and follow-up.

GENDER DIFFERENCES (Doyal 1998)

- Women have less access than men to a whole variety of economic and social resources.
- Men and women will be exposed to different health risks, both physical and psychological.
- They have access to different amounts and types of resources for maintaining or promoting their own health.
- They may have different levels of responsibility for the care of others.
- If they become ill they may have very different strategies for coping.
- They may define their symptoms in different ways, will probably look for help from different sources and could respond very differently to treatment.

GENDER

(All statistics from McPherson & Waller (1997) unless otherwise specified.)

- More males are born than females; in 1996 in the UK there were 376 000 boys compared with 357 000 girls (McPherson & Durham 1998).
- Women have a longer life expectancy than men: 74 years for men and 79 years for women.
- The most common cause of death in women is cancer (Table 1.1).

The ten commonest cancers for women in 1988 were as shown in Table 1.1 (McPherson & Waller 1997).

Table 1.1 Causes of death from cancer in women

Site	Percentage of total
Breast	25
Skin (non-melanoma)	11
Lung	10
Colon	8
Ovary	4
Rectum	4
Stomach	3
Cervix	3
Uterus	3
Bladder	2

Table 1.2 Cause of death with age

Cause	Before age 25	Before age 50	Before age 75
Breast cancer	1 in 200 000	1 in 200	1 in 30
Lung cancer	1 in 500 000	1 in 800	1 in 40
Heart attack	1 in 100 000	1 in 700	1 in 14
Stroke	1 in 40 000	1 in 500	1 in 35
Accidental death	1 in 400	1 in 200	1 in 100

- Rates of lung cancer are rising in women.
- In younger age groups women smoke more than men.
- Women smokers are less likely to give up than men.
- More women are obese than men: 16% of women, compared with 13% of men, are obese.
- Women are less physically active than men: only 57% of women take some regular exercise, whereas 72% of men take some exercise.
- Heart disease and stroke are the next most common cause of death after cancer.
- Cause of death changes significantly with age (Table 1.2).
- Women have more consultations with GPs than men, much of the disease being gender related: i.e. of all consultations in the 25–44 age group, consultations for genitourinary problems for women comprised 26% compared with 2.5% for men.
- Women consult more for
  - endocrine/nutritional/metabolic diseases
  - diseases of the blood and reproductive organs
  - mental disorders
  - diseases of the circulatory system

- genitourinary disorders
- muscular and connective tissue disorders.
- Men, on the other hand, consult more for
  - accidents
  - poisoning
  - violence.
- Women and men have similar consultation rates for
  - infectious and parasitic diseases
  - diseases of the nervous system (excluding mental disorders)
  - diseases of the respiratory system
  - disorders of the digestive system and of the skin.
- Women are prescribed more medication than men.

(McPherson & Waller 1997)

Nursing issues

Spend some time thinking about the following:

- awareness of the effect of social and economic factors on health
- knowledge of inequalities in health by availability and accessibility, real and perceived, of services and resources
- awareness of how living and working conditions can impose severe restrictions on an individual's ability to choose a healthy lifestyle
- knowledge of local social and economic profile
- knowledge of local and national information, resources and organizations
- awareness of local and national policy in social and health services.

Key points

- Factors that have improved the health status of women include:
  - better nutrition
  - improved housing and sanitation
  - public health measures
  - more effective contraception
  - safer childbirth
  - introduction of antibiotics
  - treatment of anaemia.

- Restricted access to contraception, maternal and child health may contribute to the higher prevalence of risk factors, e.g.:
  - early anFd unwanted childbearing
  - insufficient spacing between births
  - higher parity.

- These factors influence infant mortality rates and the health and well-being of mothers.

REFERENCES

Doyal L 1998 Introduction: women and health services: In: Doyal L (ed) Women and health services. Open University Press, Buckingham
McPherson A, Durham N 1998 Woman's Hour book of health. BBC Books; London, Ch 11
McPherson A, Waller D 1997 Women's health and its controversies – an overview. In: McPherson A, Waller D (eds) Women's health, 4th edn. Oxford University Press, Oxford, Ch 1
Whitehead M 1992 The health divide. Penguin, London

RACE, ETHNICITY AND HEALTH

ETHNICITY

Ethnicity may be defined as the cultural practices and outlooks that characterize a given group of people. It differentiates one group from another, by:

- language
- ancestry
- religion
- a common history
- shared cultural practices (e.g. dietary habits, style of dress).

Ethnic differences are totally learned and have nothing to do with genetic inheritance (Jones 1994). Stereotyping the behaviour and needs of ethnic groups is a form of discrimination.

RACE

Race may be defined as the physical or biological characteristics of individuals (e.g. skin tone, hair colour). It has, however, acquired a social and cultural meaning beyond physical appearance. Social meanings of inferiority and superiority have been attached to sets of physical characteristics. There are almost no systematic differences between racial groups (Jones 1994).

HEALTH AND RACE (Douglas 1998)

Most health research on black and minority ethnic communities is largely based on the assumption that there are biological differences between different 'races'. Little attention has been paid to factors differentiating individuals placed arbitrarily within particular categories. Ethnicity is influenced by:

- country of origin
- area of residence
- socio-economic status
- gender
- length of residence in Britain.

There appear to be significant differences in disease patterns between ethnic groups, but this does not take into account:

- genetic and biological differences
- environmental, geographical and cultural influences.

Social and cultural explanations should be used appropriately. They should *not* be used to:

- 'lump' together a group while ignoring religion, ethnicity, class and gender
- obscure the importance of material factors.

HEALTH ISSUES

Higher mortality rates for black and minority ethnic groups are generally concentrated in lower social classes, and in semiskilled and unskilled occupations. These groups are vulnerable to the health disadvantages associated with low income, poor housing, etc. (Jones 1994). There is, however, a higher incidence of specific diseases among certain communities. See Box 1.1 for examples.

There are rapidly developing health needs as there are fresh waves of immigrants from 'new' areas (e.g. eastern Europe). Immigrants are frequently perceived as bringing disease with them and then spreading it around indiscriminately.

Box 1.1 Incidence of diseases amongst ethnic communities (Whitehead 1992)	
Immigrants from Africa and the Caribbean	High mortality from TB, hypertension and stroke, diabetes (Caribbean only), liver cancer and maternal conditions
Immigrants from Indian subcontinent	High mortality from liver cancer, ischaemic heart disease and diabetes

SOCIAL ISSUES

- There can be difficulties for the children of 'mixed' parentage, such as:
  - conflicting health beliefs of the parents and wider family
  - conflicting cultural views on parenting and childrearing.
- Black women in the UK are more likely than their white counterparts (Douglas 1998):
  - to live in poor housing
  - to have low-paid jobs
  - to do part-time or shift work, especially working at night
  - to work outside the home while bringing up a family
  - to be caring for other relatives
  - to be exposed to occupational health hazards
  - to have an unemployed partner
  - to be told that they have to have a hysterectomy than to have alternative options discussed.

The following issues need to be taken into account when reviewing services for people from ethnic minorities:

- their previous experience of services
- their perceptions of health and well-being
- presentation of illness
- lifestyle and cultural practices
- differing patterns of disease
- use of alternative medicine.

Some health promotion activities can be targeted at the minority of an ethnic group, at the possible expense of the majority; for example concentrating on sickle cell disease, which affects a small minority, and ignoring lifestyle interventions that can affect the majority, such as reducing the risk of the consequences of hypertension and diabetes.

The age profile of the minority ethnic community is younger than the rest of the British population: 20% of the white population are aged 60+; 5% of minority communities are aged 60+. This must be taken into account when assessing health needs (Victor 1995).

Considerations when promoting health:

- 5% of the population of Great Britain are from ethnic minorities

- 50% of the ethnic minority population have been born in the UK
- it may be necessary to distinguish between the migrant and native-born components of minority communities since there may be different needs and expectations (Victor 1995).

The following factors should be borne in mind in relation to the uptake of health services (Royal College of Nursing 1996a):

- Access, e.g.
  - local awareness of services
  - time and place
  - use of trained advocates and interpreters
  - use of information and leaflets in local community languages.
- Acceptability, in that the service should take into consideration the cultural and religious values of the minority ethnic community, e.g.
  - female health care professionals
  - dietary requirements
  - traditions of death
  - use of contraception.
- Appropriateness, e.g.
  - issues about screening for genetic disorders to which only a particular group is more vulnerable
  - dietary advice and provision which takes into account cultural and religious background
  - health education which is relevant to user's cultural and religious background.

MENTAL HEALTH

Black and ethnic minority people are also more likely to be disadvantaged in terms of their mental health than the rest of the population. They are more likely to be:

- detained under the Mental Health Act
- diagnosed as suffering from schizophrenia or other forms of psychotic illness
- detained in locked wards
- regarded as 'dangerous' and treated accordingly, often leading towards gross over-representation in secure settings (Royal College of Nursing 1996b).

Alternatives to hospital admission are less likely to be offered to all minority ethnic groups (Royal College of Nursing 1996b). Asian women are three times more likely to commit suicide than other groups (Kay et al 1997).

Nursing issues

Spend some time thinking about the following:

- understanding the importance of demonstrating respect for all by carrying out holistic care and by not defining needs solely as ethnic or black issues
- awareness of discrimination of patients and colleagues on grounds of race or ethnicity
- awareness of local equal opportunities policy, this being applicable to both staff and patients
- appropriate use of trained advocacy and interpreting services
- understanding the importance of resisting forming any assumptions or stereotyping behaviour and needs
- knowledge of ethnic monitoring systems
- understanding the importance of accessing training to improve communication skills and to work effectively with patients from all ethnic groups.

Key points

- 'Minority', 'ethnic', or 'ethnic minority' is used to describe any group of people who:
  - share a cultural heritage
  - are not part of the majority (i.e. the indigenous population)
  - may experience varying degrees of discrimination (Donovan 1984).
- It can be misleading to group all members of ethnic minorities together into one disadvantaged group (Whitehead 1992).

REFERENCES

Donovan J 1984 Ethnicity and health: a research review. Social Science and Medicine 19: 663–670

Douglas J 1998 Meeting the health needs of women from black and minority ethnic communities. In: Doyal L (ed) Women and health services. Open University Press, Buckingham, Ch 4

Jones L 1994 Race, ethnicity and health. In: The social context of health and work. Macmillan Press, Basingstoke, Ch 8

Kay R, McPherson A, Waller R 1997 The role of primary health care in promoting the health of women. In: McPherson A, Waller D (eds) Women's health, 4th edn. Oxford University Press, Oxford, Ch 2

Royal College of Nursing 1996a Contracting for race and health equality: a guide for the nursing profession. RCN, London

Royal College of Nursing 1996b Race, ethnicity and mental health: the nurse's responsibilities. Issues in Nursing and Health 31. RCN, London

Victor C 1995 Inequalities in health and health promotion. In: Pike S, Forster D (eds) Health promotion for all. Churchill Livingstone, Edinburgh, Ch 12
Whitehead M 1992 The health divide. In: Townsend P, Davidson N (eds) Inequalities in health, 2nd edn. Penguin, London, Ch 2

FURTHER READING

Doyal L (ed) 1998 Women and health services: an agenda for change. Open University Press, Buckingham
Whitehead M 1992 The health divide. Penguin, London

WOMEN AND DEPRESSION

DEPRESSION

Depression is a mental state of varying duration, characterized by feelings of sadness, rejection, apathy, hopelessness, and/or withdrawal (Edge & Miller 1994). It can be so severe that those suffering from it may feel that life is not worth living.

There are two main types of depression: endogenous and exogenous.

Causes

Endogenous depression may be caused by:

- a reduction in one or more neurotransmitter, e.g.:
  - monoamines
  - serotonin
  - dopamine
- hormonal influences, e.g. Cushing's syndrome
- electrolyte changes
- vitamin B_{12} deficiency (Oliver 1993)
- a reduction in the secretion of melatonin (the hormone secreted by the pineal gland) which is thought to be implicated in seasonal affective disorder (SAD).

Exogenous (reactive) depression may be caused by life events, e.g.:

- bereavement
- financial insecurity
- unemployment
- relationship difficulties
- housing problems.

Why does it happen?

- Predisposing factors – that increase vulnerability or make it more likely that the person will develop the illness in the future.
- Precipitating factors – that trigger the illness, such as injury, bereavement or redundancy.
- Maintaining factors – that keep the illness going and prevent the person from getting better, such as chronic pain, poor social support or low self-esteem (Armstrong 1998).

Symptoms

The symptoms for both types of depression are similar:

- feelings of unhappiness that don't go away
- losing interest in life
- becoming unable to enjoy anything
- finding it hard to make even simple decisions
- feeling utterly tired
- feeling restless and agitated
- losing appetite and weight (some people do the reverse and put on weight)
- difficulty in sleeping
- waking up earlier than usual
- going off sex
- losing self-confidence
- feeling useless, inadequate and hopeless
- avoiding other people
- feeling irritable
- feeling worse at a particular time of day, usually mornings
- thinking of suicide – this is very common in depression and is much better talked about than ignored (Royal College of Psychiatrists 1996).

Incidence (Graham-Jones & Duxbury 1997)

Depression is present in 5% of attenders in general practice. It is twice as commonly diagnosed in women as men. The incidence is higher in first-degree relatives of those who have had depression. Women have a 10–25% lifetime risk. Depression is commonly associated with a physical illness which may delay diagnosis.

Women present with symptoms of anxiety and depression twice as often as men. This is due to the following factors:

- Women are differently conditioned to seek help; it is seen as more socially acceptable for women to discuss their psychological problems.
- If symptoms are too severe to cope normally, women are increasingly asking for help from doctors or seeking medication and counselling.
- Men tend to become even less communicative, and to turn to alcohol and violence.

A number of factors have been identified as indicators for increased vulnerability to depression amongst urban women:

- loss of mother before age 11
- being from a working-class background
- having three or more children under the age of 14 at home
- being unemployed
- lack of a confiding, intimate relationship with spouse (Graham-Jones & Duxbury 1997).

POSTNATAL DEPRESSION

There is a spectrum of depression that occurs in postpartum women (Clare 1994):

- 65–90% of women will experience brief episodes of emotional lability, irritability and tearfulness 2–3 days postpartum; this is known as the 'baby blues' and resolves spontaneously in a few days.
- Postpartum psychosis occurs once in every 500–1000 births; the onset is usually within the first 2 weeks following delivery; in addition to the classic features of an affective psychosis, disorientation and confusion are often noted; a severely depressed woman may have delusions that the baby is deformed or evil, and try to harm it and herself; the response to speedy treatment is generally good; the recurrence rate for a depressive illness at a subsequent puerperium is 15–20%.
- Less severe depressive disorders occur in the first postpartum year in 10–20% of mothers; most recover after a few months; social and psychological factors are important but the underlying aetiological factor is unknown.

Women with severe postnatal depression will need to be treated as in-patients.

Intervention

Treatment for depression can involve one or more of the following:

- 'talking' treatment from an appropriate counsellor, psychologist or psychotherapist
- antidepressants.

Most depression is managed in primary care. Many general practices have counsellors, psychologists or psychotherapists as part of the team, while increasing numbers of general practices have seen the benefits of carers' groups and welfare benefits advisers, in addition to counsellors etc. Health visitors have a significant role to play in supporting mothers. Box 1.2 suggests how depression and its treatment can be explained to the patient.

Box 1.2   Depression and its treatment (Jackson et al 1997)

Explanation of depression

- a common illness
- treatable, with a good outcome
- has a biochemical basis
- dispel the stigma of mental illness
- antidepressants are not addictive.

Negotiate a treatment plan

- pills for symptoms
- talk for problems.

Nursing issues

Spend some time thinking about the following:

- awareness of the incidence of depression
- improved recognition of those who may be suffering from a depressive illness
- knowledge of the symptoms and precipitating factors
- appreciation of the impact of depression on the woman and her family – occasionally there may be a child protection issue
- knowledge of different types of treatment used in own locality
- awareness of the importance of management by the *most appropriate* professional (e.g. this may be a health visitor or nurse, supported by a counsellor or psychologist)
- good knowledge of national and local information, resources and self-help groups
- sensitive awareness of possible cultural differences in the presentation, diagnosis and acceptance of the condition
- awareness of the importance of 'alternative' therapies for some.

> **Key points**
>
> - There is a strong association between environmental events and patterns of emotional disorders (Graham-Jones & Duxbury 1997). The onset of depression is usually gradual; there is rarely a sudden onset.
> - Health visitors have devised schemes, antenatally, to identify those at higher risk of developing postnatal depression.
> - Early intervention, usually in the form of increased support, can be highly effective.
> - The incidence of depression amongst young mothers is now emerging as a major contributing factor in the occurrence of psychiatric disturbance in childhood, particularly in single-parent families (Oliver 1993).

REFERENCES

Armstrong E 1998 Depression in primary care. Primary Health Care 8 (3): 17–24

Clare AW 1994 Psychological medicine. In: Kumar P, Clark M (eds) Clinical medicine, 3rd edn. Saunders, London, Ch 19

Edge V, Miller M (eds) 1994 Health promotion for women. In: Women's health care. Mosby, St. Louis, Ch 14

Graham-Jones S, Duxbury F 1997 Emotional disorders. In: McPherson A, Waller D (eds) Women's health, 4th edn. Oxford University Press, Oxford, Ch 17

Jackson G, Kassianos G, Koppel S et al 1997 Depression: a guide to its recognition and management in general practice. Consensus guidelines from Neurolink, Tunbridge Wells

Oliver R 1993 Psychology & health care. Baillière Tindall, London, Ch 1, Ch 3

Royal College of Psychiatrists 1996 Depression. Leaflet in Defeating Depression Campaign. London

FURTHER READING

Armstrong E 1998 Depression in primary care. Primary Health Care 8(3): clinical update

Graham-Jones S & Duxbury F 1997 Emotional disorders. In: McPherson A and Waller D (eds) Women's health, 4th edn. Oxford University Press, Oxford, Ch 17

PATIENT RESOURCES

Leaflets from: The Royal College of Psychiatrists, 17 Belgrave Square, London SW1X 8PG, UK.

Information about self-help groups and other support from: Depression Alliance, 35 Westminster Bridge Road, London SE1 7QB, UK. Tel.: 020 7633 9929

POVERTY AND WOMEN'S HEALTH

The link between poverty and health status has been much debated. What is clear is that women are more likely than men to suffer poverty and its effects. The health divide between those who are poor and those who are more affluent continues to widen. Those in lower socio-economic groups:

- have higher death rates in almost all areas
- experience more sickness and ill-health throughout their lives
- have lower life expectancy
- have higher rates of stillbirth and neonatal death
- may experience a poorer provision of services in more deprived areas
- have a much lower uptake rate of preventive services (Whitehead 1992).

Depression (see p 10) is an example of an illness where there is clear evidence of its disproportionate effects on women from lower socio-economic groups. There is:

- a higher incidence of depression in women from lower socio-economic groups
- more depression in women who are unemployed
  - and these women are less likely to consult their GP, and much less likely to be referred to a psychiatrist (McPherson & Waller 1997).

Age also affects the social, economic and health status of women:

- Women aged over 65 years represent 38.4% of the population.
- Half of women aged over 65 are widowed, with most living alone.
- Most older women are solely reliant on the state pension.
- Older women are more likely to suffer from disabling conditions, so requiring help from the community or from social services (Arber 1998).

THE EFFECTS OF POVERTY ON HEALTH (Graham 1998)

One in three mothers in Britain is working to meet health responsibilities on incomes below the European Union poverty line. Those living in poverty are:

- more likely to live in substandard housing
- more likely to work in a less healthy environment
- more likely to live in a high-risk environment
- more likely to have a diet high in fat and sugar, low in dietary fibre and most minerals and vitamins.

The number of households with children living in poverty is rising significantly; in 1976 there were 1.8 million households with children under the age of 16 in all households below the poverty line; this number trebled to 5.5 million by 1991. The majority of families on income support comprise lone mothers and their children. The majority of women in lower socio-economic groups are cigarette smokers. Health-promoting activities largely focus on changing health behaviour, rather than tackling the link between poverty and ill health. This is not necessarily helpful or appropriate. These health promotion activities are usually in relation to:

- diet (especially content)
- smoking
- alcohol consumption.

Local initiatives have been set up to encourage community self-help and to address neighbourhood priorities, e.g.:

- food co-ops
- tenant associations
- shared-transport schemes
- bartering schemes
- credit unions
- mothers' groups
- benefits advisers.

GOVERNMENT INITIATIVES

Radical initiatives need to address the root causes of poverty-related ill-health, e.g.:

- housing
- education
- transport
- employment
- environment
- agriculture/food policy.

Poverty disproportionately affects women and their families, and the choices they can make around where they live, what services are available in their locality and what they eat.

REFERENCES

Arber S 1998 Health, ageing and older women. In: Doyal L (ed) Women and health services. Open University Press, Buckingham, Ch 3

Graham H 1998 Health at risk: poverty and national health strategies. In: Doyal L (ed) Women and health services. Open University Press, Buckingham, Ch 1

McPherson A, Waller D 1997 Women's health and its controversies – an overview. In: McPherson A, Waller D (eds) Women's health, 4th edn. Oxford University Press, Oxford, Ch 1

Whitehead M 1992 The health divide. Penguin, London

2

Promoting health

HEALTH PROMOTION

Health is not merely the absence of illness or disease; however, there is no agreement on what is meant by health. Social class, gender, ethnic origin and occupation will affect an individual's concept of health (Naidoo & Wills 1994). Health is a state of being that is subject to wide individual, social and cultural interpretation (Jones 1994).

The terms health promotion and health education are often used interchangeably. Health promotion, however, encompasses far more than health education.

HEALTH EDUCATION

Health education aims to prevent disease by changing individual behaviour. The Department of Health (1992) in *The Health of the Nation* set targets for these behavioural changes to be achieved, by ensuring that people had the means to make informed choices in the adoption of a healthy lifestyle. Some suggest that there may be elements of persuasion and coercion in these strategies (Naidoo & Wills 1994).

A more recent Green Paper, *Our Healthier Nation* (Department of Health 1998), sets out two key aims:

- to improve the health of the population as a whole by increasing the length of people's lives and the number of years people spend free from illness; *and*
- to improve the health of the worst off in society and to narrow the health gap.

The Government suggests that there is a 'third way' to achieve good health, that falls between the old extremes of individual victim blaming and nanny state social engineering.

The prevention of ill-health in health education is usually described as primary, secondary and tertiary prevention (Box 2.1).

HEALTH PROMOTION

Health promotion, on the other hand, looks beyond the individual to his or her whole community and environment. Thus, health education could be described as the individual approach and health promotion the structural approach (Naidoo & Wills 1994).

Box 2.1 Prevention of ill-health in health education		
Primary	aimed at healthy people: to prevent ill-health and improve quality of health and life	e.g. immunization, cervical screening, contraception, accident prevention, hygiene
Secondary	aimed at those with a reversible illness, to restore health	e.g. stopping smoking, dietary changes, compliance with medication
Tertiary	aimed at those with irreversible conditions, to limit complications and maximize potential	e.g. rehabilitation after stroke, support for those with chronic conditions such as diabetes, asthma, emphysema

In 1984 the World Health Organization (WHO) attempted to define health promotion as:

the process of enabling people to increase control over, and to improve, their health. To reach a state of complete physical, mental and social well-being, an individual or group must be able to identify and to realize aspirations, to satisfy needs, and to change or cope with the environment.

1. It involves the population as a whole in the context of everyday life.
2. It is directed towards action on the causes and determinants of health to ensure that the total environment, which is beyond the control of individuals, is conducive to health.
3. It combines diverse, but complementary, methods or approaches, including communication, education, regulation, fiscal measures, organizational change, community development and spontaneous local activities against health hazards.
4. It is aimed particularly at effective public participation, supporting the principle of self-help movements and encouraging the health of the community.
5. Health professionals, especially those in primary health care, have an important role in nurturing and enabling health promotion.

Naidoo & Wills (1994) identify five approaches to health promotion:

1. Medical (expert-led with a passive client, e.g. identifying those at risk of disease), i.e. taking a blood pressure.

2. Behaviour change (expert-led with a dependent client, e.g. encouraging individuals to take responsibility for their own health and choose healthier lifestyles), i.e. encouraging dietary changes to support a supposed healthier lifestyle.
3. Educational (may be expert-led and involve the client in negotiation, e.g. increasing knowledge and skills about healthy lifestyles) i.e. supporting and facilitating a stop-smoking group.
4. Empowerment (health promoter is facilitator and the client is empowered, e.g. working with clients or communities to meet their perceived needs), i.e. a health visitor facilitating a mother and baby group.
5. Social change (the focus is at the policy or environmental level, e.g. addressing inequalities in health based on class, race, gender, geography), i.e. encouraging support of the Carers' Group, which is lobbying both local and national organizations.

HELPING PEOPLE CHANGE

To be able to help people to change their behaviour it is important to understand that they go through a number of stages in the process. Health professionals should bear this in mind when promoting health.

The Stages of Change Model (Prochaska & DiClemente 1984) identifies a six-stage cycle in this process:

Nursing issues

It is necessary for practitioners to:
- possess the necessary knowledge, skills and attitudes to communicate effectively
- have knowledge of the different approaches to health promotion
- understand the role of beliefs, attitudes and values in health-related problems (their own and those of their patients/clients)
- recognize one's own health beliefs and needs, and their effect on others
- understand influences on health
- have knowledge of local and national information, resources, groups, etc.

A possible nursing intervention could be teaching a patient with diabetes how he or she may control the condition by diet alone.

1. precontemplation of change
2. contemplation
3. decision to change (may return to contemplation)
4. action – changing
5. maintaining the changed behaviour
6. relapsing to the previous behaviour (the cycle can start again, although this stage does not always occur).

HEALTH PROMOTING ACTIVITIES

These include the following:

- sexual and reproductive health services
- screening programmes
- rehabilitation programmes
- carers' groups
- money/debt advisers
- stress management programmes
- early intervention with those at risk of postnatal depression
- working with local schools
- Look After Yourself programmes
- sharing knowledge with community groups
- joining national groups.

Key points

- Much of what is done in the name of health promotion is, in fact, health education; i.e. encouraging the take-up of preventive services which are aimed at limiting ill-health.
- Health promotion is about making the healthy choice the easier choice.
- It may take several attempts.
- You need to respect others' health priorities and acknowledge a person's right to refuse advice on lifestyle or behaviour.
- The process of change will only start when the time is right.

REFERENCES

Department of Health 1992 The health of the nation. HMSO, London
Department of Health 1998 Our healthier nation: a contract for health. Stationery Office, London
Jones LJ 1994 The social context of health and health work. Macmillan, Basingstoke, Ch 1
Naidoo J, Wills J 1994 Health promotion: foundations for practice. Baillière Tindall, London

Prochaska J, DiClemente C 1984 The transtheoretical approach: crossing traditional foundations of change. Irwin, IL
Tannahill A 1985 What is health promotion? Health Education Journal 44: 4
World Health Organization 1984 Report of the working group on concepts and principles of health promotion. WHO, Copenhagen

RESOURFCES

Health Education Authority, 30 Great Peter Street, London SW1, UK.
Tel.: 020 7222 5300

SCREENING

Screening of a healthy or 'well' person is, in fact, screening for a disease or illness. There are 10 principles for screening, all of which should be addressed before screening activities can be described as being a programme, rather than an *ad hoc* reaction to local or personal needs.

PRINCIPLES FOR SCREENING (Wilson & Junger 1960)

1. The condition should pose an important health problem.
2. The natural history of the disease should be well understood.
3. There should be a recognizable early stage.
4. Early treatment should be more beneficial than that at a later stage.
5. There should be a suitable screening test.
6. The test should be acceptable to the population.
7. There should be adequate facilities for the diagnosis and treatment of abnormalities detected.
8. For diseases of insidious onset (such as cervical cancer), screening should be repeated at intervals determined by the natural history of the disease.
9. The chances of physical/psychological harm must be less than the benefits.
10. Cost should be balanced against the benefits it provides.

More simply:

- The test should
  - have high sensitivity (will identify all positive cases)
  - high specificity (has a low false positive rate)

– be safe, cheap, simple and reliable.
- The results should be able to affect clinical management.
- There should be treatment for truly positive cases with proven clinical effectiveness.
- It should be easy to implement a workable programme. Screening should do more good than harm. Screening is targeted at the whole of a specific population, age or ethnic group.

If there is a policy about a particular condition, screening is offered to all, not just to those who are judged to be at risk.

Barriers to take-up of screening

Highly publicized failures in screening programmes, especially concerning cervical screening, have made many women question its worth. Other barriers to the take-up of screening include:

- lack of knowledge about the availability of the screening procedure
- embarrassment about the procedure, especially with cervical screening
- fear of pain with the procedure, especially with mammogram
- fear of the result
- fatalism: 'what will be will be'
- lack of confidence in the service being offered
- conviction of not being at risk.

Failures in screening programmes may be due to:

- failure to include all relevant population
- inadequately trained personnel
- inadequate or insufficient information about programme

Nursing issues

There is a need for:

- understanding of the principles of screening
- knowledge of the condition being screened
- ability to give accurate information about the whole process
- an understanding of the implications for how and when results are given
- understanding the level of anxiety and fear that many women have
- awareness of ethical, cultural and moral issues around screening.

- inability to reach quality standard
- too high false positive/negative rate
- failure of communicating results and fail-safe follow-up (the systems that ensure that a woman with an abnormal smear does not get 'lost').

CERVICAL SCREENING

- Procedure used is cervical smear.
- 1500 women die each year from cervical cancer (down from 2000 in 1990) (NHSCSP 1997).
- Offered to all sexually active women aged 20–64 years.
- Screening can continue after this age if requested.
- Screening interval 3–4.5 years.
- Invitation usually by Health Authority (HA) lists of women registered with GPs.
- Can be carried out in a number of settings.
- Can be performed by a variety of clinicians.
- Pre-cancerous changes can be detected and effectively treated.
- 85% of women in England and Scotland have been screened in the previous 5 years (DOH 1997). (See also p. 35.)

BREAST SCREENING

- Procedure used is mammogram (X-ray).
- 14 000 women die each year from breast cancer (Cancer Research Campaign 1996).
- Offered to all women aged 50–64 years, to be extended to women aged 65–70 (DoH 2000).
- Screening can continue after this age if requested.
- Screening interval 3 years.
- Invitation exclusively through HA lists of those women registered with GPs.
- Carried out in small number of dedicated centres (and some mobile units).
- Small number of dedicated clinicians.
- Cancers can be identified at an earlier stage, theoretically improving treatment outcomes.
- The current service will be upgraded by offering two view mammography, leading to an estimated 40% improvement in detection rates (DoH 2000).

- Some believe that the outcome is unaffected by screening.
- There is a 75% uptake.

Breast cancer screening can be carried out through other means. Some hospital breast departments have an early diagnostic unit. However, this is available only to some of those at high risk, having a strong family history and there is usually strict entry criteria into any screening programme. Some units may link up with specialist cancer genetics clinics, usually located in Regional Genetics Centres. Genetic testing can detect mutations on genes identified as *BRCA1* and *BRCA2*, which appear to be implicated in 70% of breast cancer families where there is a strong familial link.

A positive result means the woman is at high risk of developing breast cancer. A negative result does not, however, remove a woman's risk; it is estimated that only 5–10% of all breast cancers are ascribable to genetic causes (Chadwick 1997).

Some women choose to undergo radical surgery (e.g. bilateral mastectomy) because of their perceived risk of cancer (see p. 251).

OVARIAN SCREENING (Chamberlain 1995)

- Ovarian cancer is the most common cause of death from cancer of the genital tract.
- In the UK 5000 women are diagnosed with ovarian cancer each year.
- Over 4300 women die each year.

Procedures used include:

- Blood test to detect raised serum levels of CA 125, a tumour marker.
- Transvaginal scan of the ovaries
  – these are usually offered only to those thought to be at high risk.
- Combined tests (blood test and scan) are not sufficiently specific, with a high false positive rate (see p. 307).

OTHER SCREENING

- Rubella
  – blood test
  – routinely carried out during pregnancy

- should be carried out as part of pregnancy planning; if no immunity detected the woman can then be offered immunization.
- Pregnancy
  - human immunodeficiency virus (HIV) testing is routinely carried out in some antenatal clinics (see p. 170).
- Osteoporosis
  - bone density measurement using scanning machine, usually dual energy X-ray absorptiometry (DEXA) (see p. 196).
  - usually only targeted at those at risk of osteoporosis, or with established disease
  - result plots an individual's position on a graph, giving an indication of fracture risk.

Genetic screening is considered in the section on preconception issues (see p. 126).

Babies are routinely screened at birth using blood from heel-prick (Guthrie test):

- for phenylketonuria (incidence 1 in 10 000)
- for congenital hypothyroidism (incidence 1 in 4000)
- both conditions can be treated effectively once diagnosed.

Babies thought to be at risk may also be screened for sickle cell disease and trait, and thalassaemia.

Chlamydia: small scale screening is already carried out in some areas (e.g. those presenting for a termination of pregnancy). A swab is used to remove cells from the endocervix. There are recommendations for a national programme, but only targeting young women.

Issues around screening

- Consent (does the woman understand what she is consenting to, what the test is for, who is going to carry it out, how the test is done, and what risks the procedure carries?).
- Choice (there should never be any compulsion to have a test, e.g. an older mother does not have to have an amniocentesis).
- Confidentiality (who is going to know that a test has been carried out and what the result is).
- Information must be unbiased (any information given should not incorporate the personal opinion of the information-giver).

- Counselling must be non-directive (the patient/client should not be told what to do).
- Implications of the result must be discussed before the test (what is the person going to do if the result is positive? Are there any implications for employment, insurance, personal relationships or reproductive choices?)
- Is it worth doing, in terms both of cost-effectiveness and whether it is going to be of benefit to the individual?
- Do the benefits outweigh any risks for that individual?
- Who is the person going to share the results with? (They need to consider who they will tell about a difficult result, possibly friend, colleague or family.)

Think about the implications of testing for some diseases and disorders, e.g.:

- cystic fibrosis
- Huntingdon's chorea
- Down's syndrome
- spina bifida
- HIV.

REFERENCES

Cancer Research Campaign 1996 Breast cancer – UK. Factsheet 6. Cancer Research Campaign, London
Chadwick R 1997 Truth hurts: genetic testing for breast cancer may cause more harm than good. Nursing Standard 19(12): 19
Chamberlain G (ed) 1995 Gynaecological tumours. In: Gynaecology by ten teachers, 16th edn. Arnold, London, Ch 6
Department of Health 1997 Cervical screening programme, England: 1996–97. Statistical bulletin: Prepared by the Government Statistical Service
Department of Health 2000 The NHS Plan. The Stationery Office, London
NHSCSP 1997 Guidelines for Clinical Practice and Programme Management, 2nd edn. NHSCSP Publication No 8. NHS Cervical Screening Programme, Sheffield
Wilson JM, Junger G 1960 Principles and practice of screening for disease. WHO, Geneva

SELF-SCREENING

There are certain areas in screening where the responsibility for surveillance lies with the woman, e.g: body awareness; breast awareness; skin cancer.

Nursing issues

Spend some time thinking about the following:

- knowledge of health promotion issues
- enabling patients to take responsibility for self-screening
- promoting a healthy lifestyle
- encouraging self-awareness
- communication of accurate, current information
- access to resources
- knowledge of limits of own competency.

BODY AWARENESS

Encourage self-awareness so that changes in function are apparent:

- unintentional weight loss
- any unexplained bleeding from anywhere, including post-menopausal and post-coital bleeding
- change in bowel habit
- unexplained pain.

BREAST AWARENESS

- More than 90% of cancers are found by women themselves or by their partner.
- By the time a lump has been felt the disease can be well advanced.
- Breast awareness is the means by which possible disease can be identified, before there is a palpable lump.
- Breast awareness is knowledge of oneself so that anything *different* is apparent (see Box 2.2).

Box 2.2 Breast awareness	
Look in mirror for:	change in outline, shape or size of either breast; any puckering or dimpling of the skin; any change in the shape or position of either nipple, or change in existing nipple retraction or distortion
Feel the breasts: using a soapy hand in a bath or shower can make it part of routine; feel all over, without squeezing or prodding for:	unusual lumps, thickening or bumpy areas; any unusual change in the nipple e.g. discharge or eczema; any discomfort or pain, particularly if new, persistent or localized

Breast awareness, a five-point plan (Denton & Austoker 1995)

1. Know what is normal for you.
2. Look and feel.
3. Know what changes to look for.
4. Report changes without delay.
5. Attend for breast screening if aged 50 or over.

Key point
Many women are worried that they are going to 'fail' at breast awareness and miss 'the lump'. It is more enabling to say: 'You are not looking for a lump, you are looking to confirm that you are the way you usually are.' The woman is then empowered to report her findings, being able to say: 'I am familiar with my breasts and I know that something is different'.

The nurse's role

- To teach breast awareness
  - using leaflets
  - advising about timing, e.g. after a period
  - demonstrate to the woman how to use her hand e.g. not using her fingertips because everything will feel lumpy
  - advising the woman who has very small or very large breasts.
- To provide leaflets and verbal information and encouragement.
- Examination of the breasts, by the nurse, has no place in breast awareness:
  - it is not an effective screening technique
  - it could falsely reassure both the nurse and the woman.
- A few nurses have undertaken specialist training in breast palpation.

Guidelines produced by the RCN in 1995 conclude: 'We recommend that nurses do not undertake the practice of breast palpation and if requested to do so within their sphere of practice they should be supported in challenging such "instruction".' This guidance has since been further endorsed by the Chief Medical Officer and the Chief Nursing Officer (Practice Nurse 1998).

SKIN CANCER

- Identify those who may be at risk, through having damaged skin:
  - living in a sunny climate
  - having experienced episodes of sunburn
  - having an outdoor occupation (e.g. gardener or building-site worker)
  - hobbies
  - multiple moles.
- Encourage self-awareness so that any change is apparent, looking out for moles that:
  - are getting larger
  - have an irregular outline or are different colours of brown and black
  - are bigger than the blunt end of a pencil
  - itch, bleed or are sore.
- Some people will have an annual 'mole check'.
- Promote good practice in skin care and prevention of damage.

Key points

- There is no such thing as a healthy tan.
- The concept of self-screening is very frightening to some, as a result of:
  - fear when not doing it at all
  - fear of not doing it properly
  - fear of what might be found
  - fear of being falsely reassured.

REFERENCES

Denton S, Austoker J 1995 Watching for change: being breast aware. RCN Nursing Update. Nursing Standard 10(2): 3–9
Practice Nurse 1998 RCN breast advice is being ignored. News item. Practice Nurse 15(3): 118
RCN 1995 Breast palpation and breast awareness: guidelines for practice. Issues in nursing and health 35. Royal College of Nursing, London

BREAST SCREENING

Breast cancer is the most common cancer among women. More than 14 000 women die from breast cancer each year (NHSBSP

1997). The NHS Breast Screening Programme was set up to ensure that as many cancers as possible are detected as early as possible to maximixe the chance of successful outcomes in treatment. The NHS Breast Screening Programme was set up in 1988, on the recommendation of the report of the Forrest Committee (DHSS 1986). The programme relates to all women aged 50–64, and is due to be extended to women aged 65–70.

Invitation is strictly through lists held by Health Authorities of women registered with GPs. Screening takes place every three years and is carried out by X-ray (mammography) alone. It is only for asymptomatic women and is performed at dedicated centres around the country.

WHAT EVERY WOMAN SHOULD KNOW BEFORE SHE HAS HER MAMMOGRAM

- Breast screening centres have all female staff.
- Two X-rays are taken of each breast.
- The breast is pressed between the X-ray plates.
- The procedure can be very uncomfortable, but does not take long.
- Clinical examination of the breast has no part in the screening programme, since it is very difficult or impossible to feel tiny tumours and it is also not possible to have a consistent nationwide standard.

Nursing issues

Spend some time thinking about the following:

- how to provide accurate information and advice about the prevention and identification of breast cancer
- issues around screening, e.g. inclusion/exclusion criteria, value of procedure
- the impact of an abnormal result
- offering information about what to expect at each stage of the process
- the reasons for non-attendance
- how to encourage non-attenders to utilize the service
- appreciating social and cultural issues (e.g. modesty, fatalism)
- seeking knowledge of access to resources, including specialist breast care nurse
- those working in primary care have every opportunity to promote the service
- how to teach knowledge of breast awareness (see p. 30).

- There has been a reduction in the death rate from breast cancer, as a result of screening.
- How she will receive her results.
- What to expect if she is recalled – that it should be to a specialist breast unit.
- Every woman has at least a 1 in 12 chance of developing breast cancer anyway, but the earlier that the diagnosis is made then the better the outcome.
- There are false positive results.

WHERE CAN THE PROGRAMME FAIL?

As a result of:

- poor skill of the radiographer
- poor skill of the radiologist
- communication problems (not receiving appointment letter, not having fail-safe follow-up system).

QUALITY ASSURANCE

Monitoring all aspects of the programme includes:

- reliability of equipment
- radiation dosage
- administration of invitations
- accuracy of diagnosis.

BARRIERS TO TAKE-UP OF SCREENING

- Not being registered with a GP.
- Not having a postal address (e.g. homeless people, travellers).
- Communication problems (unable to read English, unable to read at all).
- Ignorance (I am not at risk).
- Fatalism (you can't do anything about it).
- Fear (of what might be found, of the procedure).
- Cultural attitudes.
- Loss of confidence in the system (reported failings in the programme).
- Cost of travel to centre or mobile unit.

Table 2.1   Statistics on breast screening (NHSBSP 1997)

	1995–96	1994–95
Women invited	1 517 033	1 507 605
Acceptance rate (%)	75.8	76.7
Women screened (invited)	1 149 911	1 156 333
Cancers detected	2807	2660

Key points

- The lower age limit was chosen on the basis that breast tissue in the pre-menopausal woman is much denser and therefore abnormalities would be less easily discernible.
- This lower age limit is under review, with a trial aimed at finding out whether annual breast screening by mammography at 40 years of age has an effect on breast cancer mortality.

REFERENCES

Department of Health and Social Security 1986 The Forrest report: breast screening. HMSO, London
NHSBSP 1997 NHS Breast Screening Programme 1997 Review

FURTHER READING

Austoker J, McPherson A, Lucassen A 1997 Breast problems. In: McPherson A, Waller D (eds) Women's health, 4th edn. Oxford University Press, Oxford, Ch 5

CERVICAL SCREENING

The aim of the cervical screening programme is to reduce mortality from cervical cancer. Cervical cancer can be identified at a pre-invasive stage. Malignant changes occur at the junction of glandular endocervical epithelium and squamous endocervical epithelium. The transformation zone (TZ) of the squamo-columnar junction is normally sited at the external os (Fig. 2.1). Exfoliated cells can be removed by scraping. This is the cervical smear test.

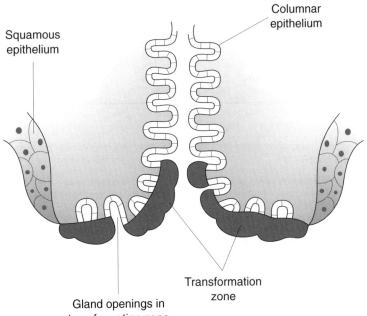

Figure 2.1   Transformation zone. The surface of the everted columnar epithelium gradually changes to squamous epithelium. This altered area, consisting of metaplastic squamous epithelium, is known as the transformation zone. In post-menopausal women there is a reduction in size of the cervix. The squamocolumnar junction and part of the transformation zone come to lie in the endocervix.

Factors that decide the position of the squamo-columnar junction are:

- Individual endogenous hormones during adolescence, puberty, the reproductive years and the climacteric/menopause (oestrogen and progesterone).
- Exogenous hormones in the form of the oral contraceptive pill and hormone replacement therapy (Padbury 1997).

The differences in the position of the squamo-columnar junction may mean that in some women it is more difficult to obtain a sample that is truly representative.

Cervical intraepithelial neoplasia (CIN) is the pre-cancerous state confirmed by histological examination of tissue removed by biopsy during colposcopy. CIN grading corresponds approximately to the cytological grading of the smear test:

- mild dyskaryosis (smear result) is consistent with CIN 1 (mild dysplasia)
- moderate dyskaryosis is consistent with CIN 2 (moderate dysplasia)
- severe dyskaryosis is consistent with CIN 3 (severe dysplasia) (see Box 2.3) Dyskaryosis (abnormal nucleus) is the term used to describe the extent of the abnormality.

WHY CARRY IT OUT?

- In the UK there are approximately 4000 new cases of cervical cancer each year.
- 1500 women died from cervical cancer in 1996 (DOH 1997).

The screening programme appears to be working because death from cervical cancer was 7.0 per 100 000 women in 1979 in

Box 2.3 Some results, their explanation and suggested action in cervical screening (Austoker & Davey 1997)		
Borderline nuclear abnormality	Nuclear changes that cannot be described as normal. There is doubt about the changes reflecting true dyskaryosis. 5% of all smears show borderline changes or mild dyskaryosis.	Repeat smear in 6–12 months. The majority of smears will be normal by this stage.
Mild dyskaryosis	Nuclear abnormalities reflecting probable CIN 1. 5% of all smears show borderline changes or mild dyskaryosis.	Repeat smear at 6 months. Many smears will return to normal by this stage. If changes persist refer for colposcopy.
Moderate dyskaryosis	Nuclear abnormalities reflecting probable presence of CIN 2. Approximately 1% of all smears show moderate dyskaryosis.	Refer for colposcopy
Severe dyskaryosis	Nuclear abnormalities reflecting probable presence of CIN 3. Approximately 0.5% of all smears show severe dyskaryosis.	Refer for colposcopy.

England and 4.1 per 100 000 women in 1995, a drop of more than 40% (DOH 1997).

WHO IS AT INCREASED RISK OF CERVICAL CANCER?

- Women in a low socio-economic group.
- Young age at first intercourse.
- Those who have had several children.
- Those who smoke.
- The woman with a history of multiple sexual partners.
- The woman who has had a sexually transmitted infection in the past.
- Those who have encountered the 'high risk' male.

There must be fail-safe systems in place to prevent women who are at risk or who have not completed treatment from being 'lost'. These systems must be understood by all those involved in the programme, at any stage.

There are guidelines aimed at maintaining the highest standards within the whole of the National Cervical Screening Programme:

- *Achievable Standards, Benchmarks for Reporting & Criteria for Evaluating Cervical Cytopathology* (NHSCSP 1995)
- *Standards & Quality in Colposcopy* (NHSCSP 1996)
- *Guidelines for Clinical Practice & Programme Management* (NHSCSP 1997)
- *Cervical Screening: Guidelines for Good Practice* (RCN 1994).

Nursing issues

Spend some time thinking about the following:

- promoting suitable health education programmes
- giving accurate information and advice about the prevention of cervical cancer
- understanding the impact of an abnormal smear
- offering appropriate help and advice at all stages of the process
- understanding the reasons for non-attendance
- encouraging non-attenders to utilize the service
- appreciating cultural issues
- maintaining regular communication with the local laboratory and colposcopy clinic, to ensure current knowledge in procedures or time for results to be sent
- regularly updating individual practice.

THE SCREENING PROGRAMME

The NHS programme was set up in 1988 to replace unco-ordinated local programmes. The programme is aimed at all women aged 20–64, with the recommendation that a cervical smear is carried out on each woman every 3 to 5 years. Invitation to screening is organized by Health Authorities, which are responsible for the computerized call and recall system, which is based on lists of women registered with GPs in that locality. Women have a choice about where their smear is carried out.

Lesbians should not be excluded from cervical screening since they:

* may have been sexually abused as a child
* may have had heterosexual sex
* can become infected with HPV though sharing sex toys.

There are misconceptions about the role of the cervical smear; it is not a diagnostic tool. A woman does not need an **extra** (i.e. more frequent) smear if she:

* starts an oral contraceptive, hormone replacement therapy, has an intrauterine device (IUD) inserted
* has a vaginal discharge, infection, genital warts
* is pregnant, post-partum, post-termination
* has had multiple sexual partners
* is a very heavy smoker (NHSCSP 1997).

By 31 March 1997 almost 85% of women aged 25–64 in England had been screened at least once in the last 5 years. In 1996–97 3.8 million women were screened, the majority after a formal invitation from the screening programme (DOH 1997).

How the programme can fail

* Poor skills of the smear-taker.
* Communication problems (not receiving letter of invitation, not attending for follow-up, not being followed-up).
* Failure by the laboratory to maintain quality standards.

The Imperial Cancer Research Fund estimated in 1996 that screening prevents between 1100 and 3900 cases of cervical cancer each year (DOH 1997).

Location

Smears can be carried out in the following locations:

- most smears are carried out in GP practices
- women can choose to go to a Family Planning or Well Woman Clinic
- smears are also carried out in various other clinics
  - gynaecology
  - colposcopy
  - genitourinary medicine (GUM)
  - antenatal
  - menopause.

Information

Before a woman has a cervical smear test, the nurse or health professional should ensure she has access to the following information (Austoker & Davey 1997):

- what condition the screening will detect, i.e. precancerous lesions
- when and how she will get the results
- the likelihood of a normal result (about 90%)
- a normal result implies low risk, not no risk
- what it means if she is recalled, e.g. an inadequate/unsatisfactory smear or an abnormal smear
- the vast majority of those who are recalled do not have cancer
- any disease detected is treatable
- she cannot have her smear while menstruating
- she should not have had intercourse (without a condom) in the previous 24 hours
- she should not have used a spermicide or lubricant in the previous 24 hours.

Inadequate smears

Five to 10% of smears are inadequate/unsuitable, due to:

- insufficient or unsuitable material present
- inadequate fixation
- poor spreading on the slide
- consisting mainly of blood and pus or inflammatory exudate.

Incidental observations and findings at the time of a cervical smear

- Infection, e.g.
  - candida
  - trichomoniasis
  - chlamydia
  (see p. 159).
- Evidence of viral infection, e.g.
  - human papillomavirus (HPV) (see p. 163)
  - herpes.
- Atrophy (cell shrinkage).
- Cytolysis (normal breakdown of cells when vaginal environment is very acidic).
- Metaplastic cells (normal cells from the transformation zone).
- Cervical ectropion (see below).
- Cervical polyps (see below).

Cervical ectropion or ectopy

- Previously termed erosion.
- Columnar epithelium from the cervical canal extends onto the surface of the cervix.
- May produce a heavy mucoid discharge.
- More common in pregnancy and in those taking the oral contraceptive pill.
- Need not be of any significance.
- Does not need to be treated unless the woman finds the discharge troublesome.

Cervical polyps

These may:

- Result from polypoid overgrowth of columnar epithelium in endocervix.
- Project through external os.
- Be found by chance at time of cervical smear.
- Offer no symptoms.
- Cause bleeding (post-coital or at examination).

They are benign, but should be removed and sent for histology.

Human papillomavirus (HPV)

- Evidence of infection with HPV may be reported on smear result.
- HPV has different strains, two of them are thought to be carcinogenic.
- HPV types 16 and 18 are present in over 80% of invasive squamous cancers of the cervix and in CIN 3.
- At present there is no acceptable system of virus typing.
- Cell changes indicate that the woman has had contact with the virus at some stage in her life.
- May not indicate active disease.
- Is not always sexually transmitted.
- Management should be based on the degree of dyskaryosis (abnormal nuclei).
- Sub-clinical warts do not need to be treated.

What prevents attendance for cervical screening?

- Not being registered with a GP.
- Not having a postal address (e.g. travellers, being homeless).
- Communication problems (e.g. unable to read, unable to read English).
- Ignorance (I am not at risk).
- Fatalism (you can't do anything about it).
- Sexual difficulties (e.g. experience of sexual assault, rape, previous difficult examination, non-consummation).
- Absolute terror of what might be found.
- Cultural attitudes.
- Cost of travel.
- Problems with childcare (some women may be made to feel unwelcome when attending for a smear with children).
- Loss of confidence in the system (high media coverage of failures in programme).

Who is excluded from the screening programme?

- Young women under the age of 20.
- Any woman who has never been sexually active.

- Women aged over 65 years (who can ask to continue with their smears if they wish).
- Women who have had a total hysterectomy for a non-malignant condition.

When should a smear be done outside the normal recall time?

Cervical pre-cancer and cancer are usually without symptoms. A smear should be done sooner if the woman reports:

- post-coital bleeding
- blood-stained vaginal discharge
- inter-menstrual bleeding
- post-menopausal bleeding.

THE PROCEDURE

- A vaginal speculum is used to visualize the whole cervix.
- Appropriate spatulae are used to wipe cells from the squamo-columnar junction (Fig. 2.2).
- A cervical brush should also be used if the transformation zone cannot be seen (this is more likely in women who are very young or post-menopausal).
- The cells are transferred to a slide and fixed.

The procedure is not usually carried out if the woman is:

- menstruating
- pregnant
- less than 12 weeks post-partum.

Nursing issues prior to carrying out procedure

Spend some time thinking about the following:

- understanding the sensitive and intimate nature of the procedure
- preserving the woman's dignity
- having the necessary skills to carry out the procedure competently and sensitively
- ensuring the woman's understanding of the reason for the test and how it is carried out
- ensuring she knows how and when she will receive the results

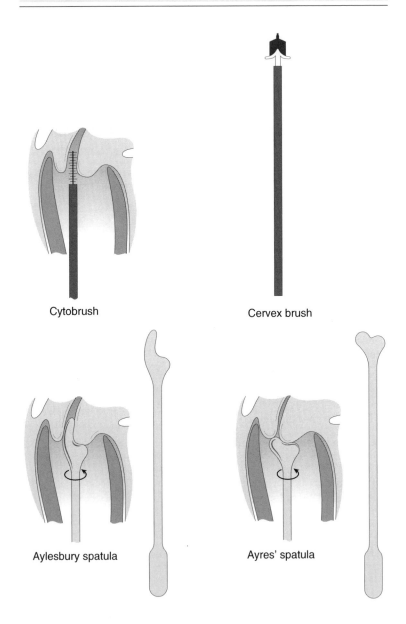

Cytobrush

Cervex brush

Aylesbury spatula

Ayres' spatula

Figure 2.2 Cervical spatulae and their position within the external os. The Ayres' spatula and the cytobrush are designed to be used together (first the spatula and then the brush), whereas the Aylesbury spatula and the Cervex brush sample both endo- and ectocervix and can be used alone.

> **Key points**
>
> - *Actinomyces* is a normal commensal of the mouth and gut.
> - The presence of actinomyces-like organisms (ALO) may occasionally show up on a cervical smear.
> - ALOs occur predominantly in women using an intrauterine contraceptive device (IUD) (see p. 118).
> - ALOs may be a marker for an increased risk of developing pelvic actinomycosis.
> - There are guidelines for the management of ALOs (Cayley et al 1998).

REFERENCES

Austoker J, Davey C 1997 Cervical smear results explained: a guide for primary care. Cancer Research Campaign, London

Cayley J, Fotherby K, Guillebaud J et al 1998 Recommendations for clinical practice: actinomyces like organisms and intrauterine contraceptives. British Journal of Family Planning 23: 137–138

DOH 1997 Cervical screening programme, England: 1996–97. Statistical bulletin: prepared by the Government Statistical Service. Department of Health, London

NHSCSP Publication No 1 1995 Achievable standards, benchmarks for reporting & criteria for evaluating cervical pathology. NHS Cervical Screening Programme

NHSCSP Publication No 2 1996 Luesley D (ed) Standards & quality in colposcopy. NHS Cervical Screening Programme

NHSCSP Publication No 8 1997 Duncan ID (ed) Guidelines for clinical practice and programme management, 2nd edn. NHS Cervical Screening Programme

Padbury V 1997 Cervical screening and abnormalities. In: Andrews G (ed) Women's sexual health. Baillière Tindall, London, Ch 11

RCN 1994 Cervical screening: guidelines for good practice. Issues in nursing and health 28. Royal College of Nursing, London

FURTHER READING

Cook R 1997 Cervical screening. Nursing Standard 11 (51): 40–46

McPherson A, Austoker J 1997 Cervical cytology. In: McPherson A, Waller D (eds) Women's health, 4th edn. Oxford University Press, Oxford, Ch 12

Padbury V 1997 Cervical screening and abnormalities. In: Andrews G (ed) Women's sexual health. Baillière Tindall, London, Ch 11

Quilliam S 1992 Positive smear, 2nd edn. Letts, London

RESOURCES

Haslett S 1994 Having a cervical smear. Beaconsfield Publishers, Beaconsfield

HEA 1996 Your smear test. NHS Cervical Screening

NHSCSP publications available from: NHS Cervical Screening Programme, The Manor House, 260 Eccleshall Road South, Sheffield S11 9PS, UK.

SEXUAL HEALTH

The World Health Organization (WHO), in 1975, defined sexual health as:

the integration of the somatic, emotional, intellectual and social aspects of sexual being in ways that are positively enriching and that enhance personality, communication and love; including
* a capacity to enjoy and control sexual and reproductive behaviour in accordance with a social and personal ethic
* freedom from fear, shame, guilt, false beliefs and other psychological factors inhibiting sexual response and impairing sexual relationships
* freedom from organic disorders, diseases and deficiencies that interfere with sexual and reproductive functions.

More briefly, it is: 'the enjoyment of sexual activity of one's choice without suffering or causing physical or mental harm' (Greenhouse 1994). Or, as Belfield (1997) has defined it:

Sexual health is determined by the political, social, economic, cultural and educational influences on our lives, and the ability we have to make decisions about and take responsibility for our sexual expression. Thus sexual health is a resource for living.

Talking about sex and sexual health can be very difficult. But it can be made easier by thinking about:

* one's own attitudes, and adopting a non-judgemental approach
* dealing with embarrassment. This can be done by demonstrating one's awareness of the embarrassment, normalizing it by saying that many people find it difficult to talk about intimate matters, and by ensuring that the relationship feels safe and can be trusted
* finding the appropriate language
* asking the right questions (Saunders 1993).

Never ask a question that you cannot give a reason for asking.

Sexual health promotion refers not only to providing information and clinical services, it also aims to empower and support people to make decisions and change their behaviour to meet their wants, needs and desires (RCN 1996)

Sexual health is more than sex. Sexual health includes:

* human immunodeficiency virus (HIV)/acquired immune deficiency syndrome (AIDS)
* sexually transmitted infections (STIs)

- sexuality and sexual behaviour
- contraception
- pregnancy (planned or unintended)
- sexual problems
- sex education.

The *Health of the Nation* (DOH 1992) identified HIV/AIDS and sexual health as priorities. The targets they set included:

- reducing the incidence of HIV infection
- reducing the incidence of other STIs
- reducing the number of unintended pregnancies (especially in under-16s).

Nursing issues

Spend some time thinking about the following:
- demonstrating sensitivity and respect for all
- developing knowledge of sexually transmitted infections (STIs) including human immunodeficiency virus (HIV) and means of prevention
- developing knowledge around fertility control issues
- being aware of issues around sexuality, including own, and also cultural and religious beliefs and differences
- ensuring understanding of exactly what constitutes safer sex
- awareness of issues around sexual abuse, and effects on sexual behaviour
- developing skills as to how to introduce issues of sex and sexual health
- exploring such issues as consent and confidentiality
- acceptance of those unwilling to alter their 'risky' behaviour
- good knowledge of accessibility to all sexual health services and personnel in locality, including those for young people and for those with disabilities
- acquiring the skills to take a good, sensitive sexual history.

BARRIERS TO SEXUAL HEALTH PROMOTION

- Inadequate training of health professionals.
- Embarrassment, on the part of both professional and client.
- Inadequate sex education.
- Fear of revealing ignorance.
- Categorizing those being 'at risk' or 'not at risk', and withholding information accordingly.
- Concerns about confidentiality.
- Lack of co-ordination and communication between services.
- Not having all methods of contraception available (including emergency contraception and condoms).

- No choice over the gender of the clinician.
- Not having facilities for the full range of STIs to be investigated.
- Lack of skills in addressing sexual difficulties.

Opportunities for sexual health promotion can be taken at:

- genitourinary medicine (GUM) clinic
- family planning/Well Woman clinic
- gynaecology clinic
- continence clinic
- schools – by the school nurse on a personal basis or as part of the National Curriculum
- sexual problems clinic
- abortion counselling
- cardiac rehabilitation
- primary care clinics
  - well person
  - antenatal/postnatal
  - new patient registration
  - travel advice
  - chronic disease (e.g. diabetes).

What is 'safer' sex?

Safer sex is the means of reducing the risk of getting infected with HIV or STIs through sexual contact by the following:

- limit number of sexual partners
- select your partner (i.e. find out his or her sexual history – not necessarily easy)
- avoid high-risk sexual practices (e.g. vaginal or anal intercourse without a condom, unprotected oral sex, sharing sex toys)
- use condoms of appropriate type (e.g. using stronger condoms and lubricant for anal sex)
- do not assume heterosexuals are not at risk.

The incidence of bisexuality is underestimated.

Key point

There are a few 'one-stop-shops' that provide an integrated sexual health service, with dedicated staff (Jones 1996). These clinics are part of the NHS and are funded by individual health authorities.

GUIDELINES

RCN 1994 The nursing care of lesbians and gay men: an RCN statement.
Issues in nursing and health. No 26. Royal College of Nursing
London

RCN 1996 Sexual health: key issues within mental health services. Royal College
of Nursing London

REFERENCES

Belfield T 1997 Family planning and sexual health services. In: FPA
Contraceptive Handbook, 2nd edn. Family Planning Association, London,
Ch 1

DOH 1992 The health of the nation. Department of Health, London

Greenhouse P 1994 Under one roof: setting up sexual health services for women.
Journal of Maternal and Child Health 19: 228–233

Jones M 1996 Clients express preference for one-stop sexual health shop.
Nursing Times 92(21): 32–33

RCN 1996 Sexual health: key issues within mental health services. Royal College
of Nursing, London

Saunders D 1993 Talking about sex. The Practitioner 237: 674, 676

World Health Organization 1975 Education and treatment in human sexuality:
the training of health professionals. Report of a WHO Meeting, Technical
Report Series, No 572

FURTHER READING

Carter Y, Moss C, Weyman A (eds) 1998 RCGP Handbook of sexual health in
primary care. Royal College of General Practitioners, London

Curtis H, Hoolaghan T, Jewitt C (eds) 1995 Sexual health promotion in general
practice. Radcliffe Medical Press, Oxford

Levy L 1997 Discussing sex. Lambeth, Southwark and Lewisham Health
Authority, London

WELL WOMAN CLINICS

Well Woman clinics are sessions, open to women of all ages, to
have a 'health check'. They may be provided by a woman's GP or
by her local community trust. Community clinics are open to all
women, providing a valuable service to those who could be
considered disadvantaged: for example, those who:

- are homeless
- have male GPs (where this presents a cultural or personal
  problem)

- have concerns over issues of confidentiality
- know that their GP has entrenched and extreme views around women's health issues.

WHAT IS A HEALTH CHECK?

It is an opportunity to:

- screen for risk factors
- promote the adoption of a healthier lifestyle
- enable the woman to make choices about her lifestyle.

Asking if she has any particular concerns that she wishes to discuss can be helpful at the beginning. Some reasons for attending that may be given are:

- taking advantage of routine screening procedures
- to discuss menstrual problems
- prompted by death or illness of a family member or friend or colleague
- concerns about lifestyle and risk factors
- to seek reassurance
- to explore sexual health issues
- to be taught breast awareness
- fertility problems.

Or to explore any of the following:

- sexual anxieties
- continence problems
- menopause
- eating disorders
- adolescent development
- premenstrual syndrome
- relationship difficulties
- stress.

Nursing issues

The need for the following should be borne in mind:

- specific training and counselling skills are essential
- need for awareness of health promotion issues
- knowledge of local screening services, resources, groups
- awareness of local and national guidelines
- awareness of limitations of role
- knowledge of referral criteria.

Some activities that may be undertaken at a Well Woman health check, as appropriate, may include:

- risk factor assessment through own and family history
- blood pressure
- weight and height (to calculate body mass index)
- urinalysis
- serum cholesterol (if appropriate)
- cervical smear
- information on breast awareness
- risk factor assessment from history, e.g.
  - cardiovascular disease
  - cancer
  - osteoporosis.

There are some procedures that should *not* be carried out as part of a routine Well Woman check.

Breast examination: breast examination is not a sufficiently sensitive procedure to identify cancers; nurses are rarely trained to carry out the procedure correctly; time is more effectively spent teaching and demonstrating breast awareness (see p. 30).

Pelvic examination: pelvic examination has no place at the time of a routine cervical smear in an asymptomatic woman; if the woman is symptomatic she is, by definition, no longer a well woman and should be referred, unless being cared for by a nurse with appropriate training. Routine pelvic examination cannot confirm or exclude ovarian cancer (see p. 307).

Both procedures should only be carried out by those who have undertaken specialist training. A routine electrocardiogram (ECG) is rarely of any value: it may give information about past events, but it cannot predict the future.

GUIDELINES

RCN 1995 Breast palpation and breast awareness: guidance for practice. Issues in nursing and health. No 35. RCN, London
RCN 1995 Bimanual pelvic examination: guidance for nurses. Issues in nursing and health. No 34. RCN, London

WHY DO WOMEN REALLY WANT A HEALTH CHECK?

Probably fewer than 50% of women come to a Well Woman clinic because they only want to take advantage of screening procedures, feeling in control of their health and well-being (author's unpublished data). Many fear that they or a family member is already at risk of or suffering from some illness. Some want support and help to make decisions about their lifestyle and to take control of their health.

Since sessions are largely run by nurses, who are seen as more approachable and accessible than doctors, women can be more comfortable about 'trivial' anxieties, for example: 'I did not want to bother the doctor about this, when there are so many really ill people' or 'I would feel embarrassed to tell the doctor this, do you think I need to see anyone?' (author's unpublished data)

WHAT CAN BE ACHIEVED AT A WELL WOMAN HEALTH CHECK?

- A relationship of trust can be established.
- Information can be collected and exchanged.
- An understanding of the woman's health beliefs can be gained.
- Negotiation about what issues the woman wants to deal with.
- Support and follow-up agreed (maintaining health is a continuing process).

> **Key point**
>
> Every woman has her own reason for attending a Well Woman session. It is necessary to find out her agenda at the outset.

WOMEN AND ALCOHOL

Women drink alcohol for a number of reasons (Illman 1997)

- to socialize
- to boost confidence
- to relax and promote sleep
- to cope with work, domestic and financial pressure
- to 'treat' sexual problems
- to relieve stress, boredom and loneliness
- to help cope with major life events
- to switch off.

There are significant differences between male and female alcoholics (Edge & Miller 1994)

- Women can identify a specific triggering event.
- Women begin drinking at an older age, but alcoholism progresses more rapidly.
- Women are prescribed more mood-altering drugs (e.g. tranquillizers and other psychotropic drugs), which can lead to multiple addictions, drug interactions, or cross-tolerance.
- Men tend to divorce their alcoholic wives, thereby reducing support systems.
- Women do not seem to receive as much social support as men.

'Safe' alcohol consumption for women is <21 units per week. 1 Unit is: 1 glass wine, $\frac{1}{2}$ pint beer, 1 measure spirits or fortified wine (e.g. sherry). Maximum health advantage is gained from 1 to 2 units per day. Regular consumption of 2 to 3 units per day gives no significant health risk.

Benefits from daily moderate drinking are lost with 'binge' drinking (Kay et al 1997).

One unit of alcohol is metabolized per hour, while food decreases the rapidity of absorption. Why are the limits less for women than for men?

- Women's bodies have 10% more fat than men.
- There is less fluid to 'dilute' alcohol.

Remember that units quoted are pub measures, and that measures poured at home tend to be much larger. After an episode of heavy drinking, it is advisable to refrain from drinking for 48 hours to allow tissues to recover (Kay et al 1997).

Nursing issues

Spend some time thinking about the following:

- awareness of the risks of high levels of alcohol consumption
- awareness of the signs that might indicate high alcohol consumption
- sensitive giving of accurate information about safe drinking levels
- elicit woman's own concerns and level of knowledge
- offer encouragement
- support and advice concerning associated problems
- utilize local alcohol services.

WOMEN AND DRINKING, SOME FACTS (Alcohol Concern 1997)

- 14% drink more than 14 units per week.
- 2% drink more than 35 units per week.
- Women are more likely to be abstainers.
- Women's drinking is on the increase.
- Young women drink the most and have the highest levels of alcohol dependence.
- Altogether about 28 000 to 33 000 people die each year from alcohol-related causes.
- Half a million women in Britain are dependent on alcohol.

In Britain:

- Young women are more likely to drink than older women.
- Nearly 20% of 16–24 year olds drink over 14 units per week.
- Professional women are more likely to exceed limits.
- Full-time workers are almost twice as likely to exceed sensible drinking limits as women who work part-time or not at all (Alcohol Concern 1997).

Simple interventions can be highly effective, despite drinking habits often being very hard to break. Keeping a drinking diary and agreeing to short-term goals may be the first step (Kay et al 1997). See Box 2.4 for a questionnaire about drinking habits.

Light to moderate alcohol consumption can give a protective effect against:

- coronary heart disease (CHD)
- ischaemic stroke
- cholesterol gallstones (Kay et al 1997).

Box 2.4 How to tell if you have a drink problem

- Have you ever felt you ought to **C**ut down on your drinking?
- Have people **A**nnoyed you by criticizing your drinking?
- Have you ever felt bad or **G**uilty about your drinking?
- Have you ever had a drink first thing in the morning (an **E**ye-opener) to get rid of a hangover?

Referred to as the **CAGE** questionnaire

High levels of alcohol consumption are associated with:

- hypertension

- liver cirrhosis
- cardiovascular disease
- cancers of mouth, pharynx and oesophagus.

Heavy, long-term consumption is associated with:

- mental illness
- social/interpersonal problems
- neurological disease
- liver cancer
- osteoporosis.

Excess alcohol consumption is linked with:

- rape (of women)
- assault
- relationship problems
- accidents
- drug abuse
- child abuse
- absenteeism
- divorce
- suicide.

ALCOHOL AND FERTILITY

- Heavy drinking can suppress ovulation.
- Heavy drinking in men affects quality of sperm.

Alcohol in pregnancy:

- increases risk of spontaneous second trimester abortion
- more fetal abnormalities
- heavy drinking may lead to a baby with the physical abnormalities and mental retardation of fetal alcohol syndrome.

There is little or no evidence to suggest that light drinking (two or three drinks per week) causes fetal damage (Sweet 1988; Alcohol Concern 1998).

ALCOHOL AND BREAST CANCER

The Cancer Research Campaign (1996) describes how several studies have suggested a link between alcohol and breast cancer.

The risk seems to increase in women who drink more than 3 units per day. However, the proof is inconclusive and the advice to any woman is to keep within recommended limits. These findings are endorsed by other research (Kay et al 1997).

Advice on sensible drinking can incorporate the following points:

- limit your drinking to 2 units per day
- do not drink during the day
- have alcohol-free days each week
- remember that your health can be damaged without being 'drunk'
- regular heavy intake is more harmful than occasional binges
- do not drink to 'drown your problems'.

TEN TIPS FOR CUTTING DOWN (HEA 1997)

1. Keep a drink diary.
2. Stick to the limit you've set.
3. Watch it at home (home drinks are usually larger).
4. It's OK to say no.
5. Avoid rounds (drink at your pace).
6. Pace your drinks.
7. Occupy yourself.
8. Find alternatives (for relaxation).
9. Have days when you don't drink at all.
10. Reward yourself.

DETECTING THE PROBLEM

Information may be supplied by family and others. Alcohol problems may be physical, psychological or social and may present as:

- gastrointestinal disorders
- anxiety
- depression
- work problems
- accidents.

Some people cannot cut down and so are advised to abstain. Indications for advising abstinence are:

- Absolute
  - alcohol-related organ damage
  - severe dependence (morning drinking to stop the shakes, previous failure to control)
  - significant psychiatric disorders.
- Relative
  - epilepsy
  - social factors (legal, employment, family)
  - other physical problems.

LOCAL SERVICES

Provision of local services is varied. The following services may be available (UK Alcohol Forum 1998):

- community alcohol service
- community alcohol team
- alcohol specialist psychiatrist
- specialist alcohol unit
- community psychiatric nurse (CPN) with alcohol remit.

REFERENCES

Alcohol Concern 1997 Women's drinking: facts and figures. Information Unit Factsheet 05. Alcohol Concern, London
Alcohol Concern 1998 A woman's guide to alcohol. Alcohol Concern, London
Cancer Research Campaign 1996 Breast cancer – UK. Factsheet 6. Cancer Research Campaign, London
Edge V, Miller M (eds) 1994 Health promotion for women. In: Women's health care. Mosby, St. Louis
HEA 1997 Say when ... how much is too much? Health Education Authority, London
Illman L 1997 Promoting a healthy lifestyle. In: Andrews G (ed) Women's sexual health. Baillière Tindall, London
Kay R, McPherson A, Waller D 1997 The role of primary health care in promoting the health of women. In: McPherson A, Waller D (eds) Women's health, 4th edn. Oxford University Press, Oxford, Ch 2
Sweet B 1988 Health education. In: Maye's midwifery, 11th edn. Baillière Tindall, London, Ch 18
UK Alcohol Forum 1998 Guidelines for the management of alcohol problems in primary care and general psychiatry. UK Alcohol Forum, High Wycombe

RESOURCES

Alcohol Concern, Waterbridge House, 32–36 Loman Street, London SE1 0EE, UK. Tel.: 020 7928 7377

HEALTHY LIFESTYLE

A healthy lifestyle is promoted with the intention of preventing the onset or progress of some diseases through screening procedures and by identifying risk factors for conditions and by encouraging modifying behaviour. Cigarette smoking, high alcohol consumption, poor diet and lack of exercise all contribute to deaths from cancers, respiratory disease and heart disease/stroke (Victor 1995).

Coronary heart disease is the commonest cause of death in women over 50 years. The older a woman gets the more likely she is to die of a disease of the circulatory system.

When carrying out patient/client education, there are some principles that should always be observed (Ewles & Simnett 1999):

- Say important things first.
- Stress and repeat key points.
- Give specific, precise advice.
- Structure information into categories.
- Avoid jargon, long words and long sentences.
- Use visual aids, leaflets, handouts and written instructions to back up what you say (but not instead of talking it through).
- Avoid saying too much at once.
- Ensure advice is relevant and realistic.
- Get feedback to ensure that advice and information have been understood.

Making an assessment of risk factors is the first part of promoting a healthy lifestyle. It is rare for one factor to be significant on its own. The combined effect of multiple factors is greater

---

Nursing issues

It is important for anyone promoting health to consider the following:

- ensure excellent communication skills
- gain accurate knowledge of issues
- be aware of local guidelines and resources
- have an awareness of social, cultural and emotional needs and values
- understand the principles of patient education
- provide sensitive, holistic care
- work with other team members as necessary (e.g. dietitian, smoking cessation nurse, etc.).

than the sum of the individual components (Hargrave et al 1997). See Box 2.5 for the risk factors associated with coronary heart disease.

Box 2.5   Highest risk factors associated with coronary heart disease

Modifiable
Smoking
High blood pressure
Overweight/obesity
Lack of exercise
Alcohol
Salt intake
Raised total cholesterol

Non-modifiable
Age
Gender
Genetic history

MOTIVATIONAL INTERVIEWING (Box 2.6)

This is a technique that can work well as a method of assessing an individual's risk factors and how she feels about them (Hargrave et al 1997).
The technique relies on:

- Active listening (i.e. making it clear that you are listening by means of verbal and non-verbal behaviour).
- Asking open questions, which give the patient/client an opportunity to respond however they want; there is often no correct answer (i.e. 'could you tell me how you have been managing the shopping and cooking since I last saw you?', rather than 'have you been sticking to your diet?').
- Reflecting responses (i.e. repeating back the words that the patient/client has spoken so that she may hear them more clearly).
- Picking up clues, by paying attention to the language and body-language that the patient/client uses.
- Establishing the individual's position in process of change, and how likely she is to progress to the next stage.

Box 2.6   Techniques in motivational interviewing

- establish rapport
- identify the problem: do the patient's and nurse's priorities differ?
- focus on the priority
- help the patient come to terms with any barriers to change
- negotiate and plan changes.

Lifestyle issues that you may seek to cover in motivational interviewing:

- weight
- diet
- exercise
- smoking
- alcohol
- blood pressure.

Weight

Obesity is associated with the following:

- raised blood pressure
- elevated total plasma cholesterol and triglycerides
- lower high-density lipoprotein (HDL) (a lipoprotein subfraction that transports cholesterol)
- increased insulin resistance and risk of diabetes
- increased risk of further myocardial infarct.

Fat distribution appears to be important (central obesity, measured as waist-hip ratio, is an independent risk factor) (Poulter et al 1996).

Obesity may be measured by body mass index (BMI), a formula that grades weight into bands (Box 2.7).

The formula:

$$BMI = \frac{Weight\ (kg)}{Height^2\ (m)}$$

Box 2.7 BMI grades

Less than 20	underweight
20–24.9	acceptable
25–29.9	overweight (some health risk)
30–40	obese (moderate health risk)
Over 40	severely obese (high health risk)

Dieting does not seem to work, with 98% of women who have dieted regaining the weight they had lost and often gaining more within 2 years of the weight loss. There appears to be good evidence that 'yo-yo' dieting is associated with increased morbidity and mortality (Kay et al 1997).

'Weight gain rather than weight loss is the outcome of dieting in most people' (Freeman & Newton 1993).

Messages around weight control should be positive rather than negative:

- Look at what can be done rather than what cannot.
- Concentrate on what can be increased rather than decreased (e.g. more fruit and vegetable, complex carbohydrate and exercise).

Diet

Balance of Good Health (HEA 1996) is a publication that aims to reduce confusion about the meaning of 'healthy eating'.

Dietary advice suggests increasing monounsaturated fatty acids, polyunsaturated fatty acids and complex carbohydrates.

Recommended modifications to lifestyle are:

- Salt restriction   Avoid salty foods and do not add extra salt to food during cooking or at the table.
- Potassium intake   Increase consumption of fresh fruit and vegetables.
- Weight reduction   Dietary advice.
- Exercise   Low intensity (see below).
- Alcohol   Restrict to 2 units per day.

Exercise

Regular moderate exercise can reduce blood pressure. Prolonged periods of immobility increase the risk of osteoporosis, whilst regular weight-bearing exercise can increase bone formation (NOS/RCN 1996). Regular exercise can improve general well-being and relieve stress (Kay et al 1997). Regular exercise is defined as physical activity that is taken:

- at least 3 times a week
- for at least 20–30 minutes
- at such a rate that the heart rate is increased.

Some women who have stress incontinence will benefit from being taught how to perform pelvic floor exercises (see p. 276).

Smoking

Smoking does not directly cause hypertension, but it is a significant factor in the following:

- coronary heart disease
- cerebrovascular accidents (CVA)
- peripheral vascular disease
- chronic obstructive pulmonary disease
- lung cancer
- problems associated with low-birth-weight babies.

It is also implicated as a factor in the development of osteoporosis (NOS/RCN 1996)

Alcohol (see p. 52)

Alcohol causes an acute rise in blood pressure. The effect on blood pressure is transient, with it returning to normal after a period of abstinence following a binge (Poulter et al 1996). Heavy drinking significantly increases risk of CVA, whilst moderate alcohol consumption may be cardioprotective (by increasing HDL).

The recommended maximum weekly intake for women is 21 units (see p. 53).

Blood pressure (see p. 203)

Culture and race influence the incidence of obesity, hypertension, diabetes and coronary heart disease. There is a higher than average incidence of hypertension among African–Caribbean women, diabetes among women from South Asia and coronary heart disease among women in Scotland. These may be due to genetic and dietary influences, among others (Douglas 1998, Sharp 1998).

The goals of treatment of hypertension are to achieve a systolic pressure no greater than 160 mmHg and a diastolic pressure no greater than 90 mmHg (British Hypertension Society 1997). These goals are currently under review.

REFERENCES

British Hypertension Society 1997 Management guidelines in essential hypertension

Douglas J 1998 Meeting the health needs of women from black and minority ethnic communities. In: Doyal L (ed) Women and health services. Open University Press, Buckingham, Ch 4

Ewles L, Simnett I 1999 Promoting health: a practical guide, 4th edn. Baillière Tindall, London

Freeman C, Newton R 1993 Eating disorders. In: McPherson A (ed) Women's problems in general practice, 3rd edn. Oxford University Press, Oxford, Ch 17

Hargrave P, Johnson K, Skypala I 1997 Heart health: prevention. RCN Nursing Update. Royal College of Nursing, London

Health Education Authority 1996 The balance of good health. HEA, London

Kay R, McPherson A, Waller D 1997 The role of primary health care in promoting the health of women. In: McPherson A, Waller D (eds) Women's health, 4th edn. Oxford University Press, Oxford, Ch 2

National Osteoporosis Society/Royal College of Nursing 1996 Osteoporosis resource pack. NOS, Radstock

Poulter N, Sever P, Thom S 1996 Cardiovascular disease: practical issues for prevention, 2nd edn. Whitfield, Surbiton

Sharp I 1998 Gender issues in the prevention and treatment of coronary heart disease. In: Doyal L (ed) Women and health services. Open University Press, Buckingham, Ch 6

Victor C 1995 Inequalities in health and health promotion. In: Pike S, Forster D (eds) Health promotion for all. Churchill Livingstone, Edinburgh, Ch 12

RESOURCES

British Heart Foundation, 14 Fitzhardinge Street, London W1H 4DH, UK. Tel.: 020 7935 0185.

Health Education Authority, 30 Great Peter Street, London SW1, UK. Tel.: 020 7222 5300.

3

Ethico-legal issues

Consent and confidentiality are important issues that effect all people, at all times. Assisted conception and issues around contraception and consent are of particular importance to women, significantly affecting many women each year.

ASSISTED CONCEPTION: ETHICAL ISSUES

The Human Fertilisation and Embryology Authority (HFEA) was created by the Human Fertilisation and Embryology Act (1990). The HFEA's principal tasks are to license and monitor clinics that carry out:

- in vitro fertilization (IVF)
- donor insemination (DI)
- embryo research.

The following treatments are licensed by the HFEA:

1. DI.
2. Gamete intra-fallopian transfer (GIFT).
3. IVF.
4. Intra-cytoplasmic sperm injection (ICSI).

5. IVF using donated eggs, sperm or embryos.
6. Transport/Satellite IVF.
7. Embryo freezing and storage.

Box 3.1   The HFEA's other main functions

- To keep a formal register of information about donors, treatments and children born from those treatments. This is so that children born as a result of donated eggs or sperm can find out, if they wish, something about their genetic history.
- To produce a Code of Practice which gives guidelines to clinics about the proper conduct of licensed activities.
- To publicize its role and provide relevant advice and information to patients and donors and clinics.
- To keep under review information about embryos and any subsequent development of embryos and about the provision of treatment services and activities governed by the 1990 Act and advise the Secretary of State if s/he asks about those matters. (HFEA 1997)

The HFEA also regulates the storage and disposal of gametes (sperm and eggs) and embryos. The primary aim is to safeguard all relevant interests, including those of:

- the patient
- donors
- children
- the wider public
- future generations.

Other functions of the HFEA are shown in Box 3.1. The objectives are to ensure that: 'treatment and research are undertaken with the utmost respect and responsibility' (HFEA 1997).

Each clinic must be licensed. There is an annual inspection and the accuracy and completeness of data collected from the clinics must be assured.

THE CODE OF PRACTICE (Box 3.2)

The Code is reviewed regularly and updated accordingly. The most recent revision (1997) included:

- the upper age limit for sperm donors (currently 55 years)
- the screening of donors for cystic fibrosis
- the statutory storage period for embryos (5 years, except in exceptional circumstances)

- the treatment of HIV antibody positive parents (the welfare of any potential child and the health of the couple requiring infertility treatment must be taken into account).

Reports of breaches of the Code of Practice must be investigated.

Box 3.2 Code of Practice for clinics carrying out licensed activities

Provides guidelines and standards on:
- staff and facilities
- assessment of patients and donors
- patient literature
- procedures for counselling and obtaining consent
- handling and storage of gametes and embryos
- record-keeping
- security
- complaints procedure.

RESEARCH

Research projects using human embryos must be licensed and must be shown to fulfil one of the following purposes:

- Promote advances in the treatment of infertility.
- Increase knowledge about the causes of congenital disease.
- Increase knowledge about the causes of miscarriage.
- Develop more effective techniques of contraception.
- Develop methods for detecting the presence of gene or chromosome abnormalities in embryos before implantation.

ETHICAL ISSUES

These are always being reviewed in the light of fast-moving technology. Current concerns include:

- Pre-implantation genetic diagnosis – a technique used to detect whether an embryo created in vitro is carrying a genetic defect which will give rise to a serious inherited disorder; it can also be used to determine the sex of an embryo where a family is at risk of passing on a serious sex-linked disorder.
- Payment to gamete donors – currently £15 per donation plus reasonable expenses.
- Safe cryopreservation of sperm and embryos – to prevent cross-contamination through storage with other materials.

- Cloning – is not licensed.
- Consent to sperm donation – Diane Blood eventually succeeded in obtaining her dead husband's sperm despite not having his written consent (HFEA 1997).

The HFEA also:

- Keeps a confidential register of information about donors, patients and treatments.
- Gives advice and information to licensed clinics.
- Gives information to people seeking fertility treatment, to donors and to people needing to store their sperm, eggs, or embryos as well as to the general public.

GUIDELINES

Transport IVF: guidelines for nurses working in units offering transport in vitro fertilisation. Royal College of Nursing, 1996.

SURROGACY

Surrogacy is the arrangement by which a fertile woman has a baby for an infertile couple. The Surrogacy Arrangements Act 1985 allows non-commercial surrogacy.

'Straight' surrogacy is when the woman is artificially inseminated with the sperm of the infertile woman's partner or an IVF procedure is carried out with the surrogate woman's egg and the sperm from the infertile woman's partner. 'Host' surrogacy is an

---

Nursing issues

Spend some time thinking about the following:

- the role of the HFEA
- awareness of the sensitivity of all ethical issues, especially concerning donated gametes
- awareness of local policy around access to assisted conception techniques
- supporting the patient and her partner with information about resources and organizations and how to choose an assisted conception clinic
- knowledge of issues around consent and confidentiality
- knowledge of issues around HIV and genetic testing.
- sperm donors are paid
- egg donors are not paid.

IVF procedure using both egg and sperm from the infertile couple, which is placed in the surrogate's uterus.

Surrogacy is a legitimate alternative treatment to childlessness, when other alternatives have been exhausted. A Parental Responsibility Agreement makes it much easier to transfer legal parenthood to the commissioning couple. Surrogate mothers can, legally, be paid 'reasonable' expenses only.

Some ethical considerations:

- What if fetal abnormalities are detected in early pregnancy?
- Who takes responsibility if the surrogate mother has medical problems as a result of the pregnancy?
- What if the child is born with a defect?
- What if the surrogate refuses to hand over the baby?

There are no 'right' answers to these questions. However, they are potential problems that should be considered before embarking on this course of action. Appropriate counselling is essential. A surrogacy arrangement is unenforcable in law. The best interests of the child are paramount (Mack & Tucker 1996, Power 1997, McHale 1998).

REFERENCES

HFEA 1997 Human Fertilisation and Embryology Authority Sixth Annual Report. London
Mack S, Tucker J 1996 Fertility counselling. Baillière Tindall, London
McHale J 1998 Reproductive choice. In: McHale J, Tingle J, Peysner J (eds) Law and nursing. Butterworth Heinemann, Oxford, Ch 11
Power M 1997 Fertility problems. In: Andrews G (ed) Women's sexual health. Baillière Tindall, London, Ch 8
RCN 1996 Transport IVF: guidelines for nurses working in units offering transport in vitro fertilisation. Royal College of Nursing, London

CONFIDENTIALITY

Nurses are expected to keep all information about patients in the strictest confidence. Confidentiality is essential to a relationship based on trust. If patients do not have confidence that information about them will be kept confidential, either they will not reveal information that is relevant to their care or they will not seek care in the first instance.

All records and other information should only be made available to those directly involved in patient care. Clause 10 of the UKCC's Code of Professional Conduct (1992) makes it clear that nurses must respect patient confidentiality and follow the common law. Confidentiality can only be breached in *exceptional* circumstances:

- on the order of a court of law
- when it is felt that disclosure of information would be in the public interest.

The common law requires that any confidence obtained in a relationship of trust should be kept private unless consent has been given for this to be disclosed (Caulfield 1997).

Nursing issues

Spend some time thinking about the following:

- ensuring there is a common understanding of what confidentiality means. This may be between
  - nurses
  - nurses and other health professionals
  - nurses and patients, and patients' relatives
  - health professionals and ancillary staff
- awareness of local confidentiality policy (see Box 3.3)
- documenting only what is necessary
- the age and condition of the woman make no difference to her right to confidentiality
- ensuring the woman's understanding of the need to share some information with other team members
- being aware of conditions under which disclosure may be necessary
- being prepared to justify any breach of confidence
- considering difficulties of a consultation where the woman is not alone (e.g. with friend, parent, partner, carer, interpreter).

Box 3.3 Statement of confidentiality

An example for primary care that may be written in the practice leaflet and displayed in the waiting room.
 'We have strict rules about confidentiality which apply to all our staff. We are especially careful that family members should not be able to learn things about each other unless consent has been given by the patient concerned. If you have worries about confidentiality please feel free to discuss it with our doctors or nurses' (Damerell & Moss 1998).

AREAS TO CONSIDER WHEN REVIEWING CONFIDENTIALITY

- Clauses in all staff contracts.
- Storage and access to notes.
- Computer access.
- Discussion in public areas.
- Overheard telephone calls.
- Security of faxes, e-mails and letters.
- Teaching students.
- Concerns of young people.
- How sensitive information is recorded.
- How results of tests are given.
- How appointments are made.
- Use of reflective journals for portfolio/course work purposes.

Key points

- A duty of confidence would be implied in a situation in which a patient discloses information to a nurse because of her or his status as a nurse.
- The nurse is obliged by both law and professional practice to keep the patient's confidence (McHale 1998).

GUIDELINES

Genetic Screening and Confidentiality (RCN 1997) suggests some questions to be asked when considering the disclosure of information:

- what would be gained?
- who would benefit?
- what harm might be caused?
- is the action justified?

Confidentiality and People Under 16

Guidance issued jointly by the BMA, GMSC, HEA, Brook Advisory Centres, FPA and RCGP, 1993. This states: 'The duty of confidentiality owed to a person under 16 is as great as the duty owed to any other person' and: 'An explicit request by a patient that information should not be disclosed to particular people, or indeed to any third party, must be respected save in the most exceptional circumstances'.

The nurse/health professional should always be able to explain to the patient exactly what information needs to be shared with other team members and why. The patient should always be asked for his or her consent to this. Some of the many areas in which confidentiality may be broken either inadvertently or deliberately include:

- Insurance medical reports (the Access to Medical Reports Act 1988 gives statutory right of access to reports compiled for the purposes of employment or insurance).

- Pre-employment reports: these may enable a prospective employer to discriminate against the patient.
- Child sex abuse: the UKCC (1996) gives guidance that disclosure of suspected child abuse is justified as being in the public interest.
- HIV status: some companies insist on pre-employment testing. Is adequate counselling given prior to testing? Should someone be informed of their partner's status? What about those working in areas of high risk to the public because of their own HIV status, e.g. an HIV positive surgeon?
- Suspected serious crime: the crime would have to be very serious for disclosure to be justified, e.g. murder or terrorism.
- Sexually transmitted infection: there is legislation restricting the disclosure of identifiable information in this area to the doctor caring for the patient, or to the person who has had the responsibility for that care delegated to them (e.g. a nurse in a GUM clinic) or to prevent the spread of the infection (McHale 1998).
- Gamete donation: the Human Fertilisation and Embryology Act 1990 places a ban on the disclosure of information concerning donors of sperm and eggs and those receiving treatment for infertility.
- Local child protection policy: awareness of local systems and procedures.

REFERENCES

BMA, GMSC, HEA, Brook Advisory Centres, FPA and RCGP 1993 Confidentiality & people under 16. BMA, London

Caulfield H 1997 Legal aspects of confidentiality. Primary Health Care 8: 28–29

Damerell A, Moss C 1998 Confidentiality. In: Carter Y, Moss C, Weyman A (eds) RCGP handbook of sexual health in primary care. Royal College of General Practitioners, London, Ch 3

McHale J 1998 Confidentiality and access to health care records. In: McHale J, Tingle J, Peysner J (eds) Law and Nursing. Butterworth-Heinemann, Oxford, Ch 7

RCN 1997 Genetic screening and confidentiality. Issues in nursing and health 44. Royal College of Nursing, London

UKCC 1992 Code of Professional Conduct. United Kingdom Central Council for Nursing, Midwifery and Health Visiting, London

UKCC 1996 Guidelines for Professional Practice. United Kingdom Central Council for Nursing, Midwifery and Health Visiting, London

FURTHER READING

McHale J, Tingle J, Peysner J 1998 Law and nursing. Butterworth-Heinemann, Oxford

CONSENT

Consent to treatment is a fundamental right. A fundamental principle of health care law and ethics is that treatment should only be given with the patient's consent (McHale 1998). Consent to treatment can be implied, spoken or written.

IMPLIED CONSENT

This involves mainly non-verbal communication, for example:

- coming to a clinic
- rolling up a sleeve for recording blood pressure or taking a blood sample
- removing clothing for a treatment or procedure.

SPOKEN, OR VERBAL, CONSENT

- Saying what she wants to have done.
- Agreeing about what she has come for.

WRITTEN CONSENT

- Given prior to surgery.
- Given prior to some treatments or procedures.

CONSENT AND YOUNG PEOPLE

'Any competent young person, regardless of age, can independently seek medical advice and give valid consent to medical treatment' (BMA et al 1993). This guidance document clarified the right of young people to consent to, or to refuse, treatment, the ability to give consent being based on maturity rather than age (see p. 71).

Nursing issues

Spend some time thinking about the following:

- accurate knowledge of the specific situation involved
- the ability to communicate effectively
- the ability to present unbiased information
- demonstrating respect for woman's level of knowledge
- respecting any decision to refuse consent
- awareness of the rights of everyone, regardless of age and intellectual capacity
- understanding that informed consent can only be given if adequate information is provided in a manner that is appropriate to that individual.

POINTS TO CONSIDER

- How much information is given.
- How the information is given.
- How the information is balanced.
- What type of language is used (too much jargon, too medical).
- Choice of words, body language (indicating distaste or unease).
- Citing advantages before disadvantages, or vice versa.
- Explaining risk in an understandable way.
- What information is withheld.
- Exchanging information.
- Ensuring information has been understood.
- Encouraging questions.
- Supporting the decision, whatever it is.
- Understanding whose decision it is.
- Awareness of any moral or ethical dimension to the decision.

There are many decisions that any woman could have to make at some stage in her life, involving issues of consent, including:

- Using emergency contraception: will it work? What are the risks?
- Using any contraception: will it work? What are the risks? Does it conflict with religious and cultural beliefs?
- Having a baby: is it the right time? Is it the right relatio ship?
- Having an abortion: is the woman being pressured by others to have or not to have the baby?
- Undergoing a screening procedure: how accurate are the results? Does a negative result mean you don't get the disease? Who reviews and checks the quality of those carrying out the screening test?
- Genetic testing: what are the implications of the result on the patient, partner and family? Would you rather not know?
- Going to a sexual health clinic: who is going to find out? How may it affect the woman's relationship with her partner?
- Immunization: are these the full facts? Is there an acceptable alternative?
- Sterilization: is it reversable? What about the young woman with a learning disability?

- Rejecting conventional therapies: what is the evidence? Is a patient categorized as difficult if she questions accepted practice?
- Refusing a Caesarean section: does it place the unborn child at risk? Is it right that the courts can sanction an enforced Caesarean section? What about the right of the mother?
- Refusing a hysterectomy: have the alternatives to hysterectomy been fully explained and explored? Is the woman aware that there may be alternatives for her?
- Requesting hormone replacement therapy (HRT): does the woman have reasonable expectations of the effects of HRT? Has she been refused HRT because the menopause is a natural event that every woman goes through or because of ignorance of the true contraindications?

Key points

- Never assume that people understand what they appear to be consenting to.
- With multiple blood tests is the patient consenting to each individual sample? What are the implications of a positive HIV test, when the patient is unaware that testing has taken place?

REFERENCES

BMA, GMSC, HEA, Brook Advisory Centres, FPA, RCGP 1993 Confidentiality & people under 16
McHale J 1998 Consent to treatment 1: general principles. In: McHale J, Tingle J, Peysner J (eds) Law and nursing. Butterworth-Heinemann, Oxford, Ch 5

FURTHER READING

McHale J, Tingle J, Peysner J 1998 Law and nursing. Butterworth-Heinemann, Oxford

---

CONTRACEPTION AND CONSENT

When considering contraception and consent it is important to remember that *all* women must have the opportunity to make an informed choice of their method for themselves (see p. 113). All information must be given in an informed, unbiased and non-directive manner. No woman will be satisfied with her method of contraception unless it is her own choice.

A young woman under 16 years may be given contraceptive advice and treatment provided that:

- it is considered to be in her best interests
- she understands the issues around what she is consenting to.

Young people under 16 are legally able to consent, on their own behalf, to any surgical, medical or dental procedure provided, in the doctor's opinion, they are capable of understanding the nature and possible consequences of the procedure: 'Any competent young person, regardless of age, can independently seek medical advice and give valid consent to medical treatment' (BMA et al 1993).

A young woman under 16 may consent to an abortion, or equally she may refuse to have an abortion.

The Children Act (DOH 1989) gave children the authority to consent to treatment and to refuse treatment.

In 1974 the DHSS issued a memorandum of guidance to doctors advising:

- contraceptive advice could be given to girls aged under 16, without telling their parents
- they should always ask the girl's permission to tell her parents.

However, in 1980 part of the memorandum was reissued emphasizing:

- the need to persuade the girl to involve the parents or guardian
- the decision whether to involve the parents or not ultimately lay with the clinician.

How this guidance was interpreted varied enormously. One clinic would refuse even to see anyone who was under 16; in another, an initial consultation would be carried out, but the young woman would be told that she would have to bring her parents to the next appointment; while in a third clinic a young woman would be enabled to fulfil her contraceptive needs, while being encouraged to involve her parents. Widespread among young people at that time was the belief that advice, let alone treatment, was not available, regardless of age.

Eventually, following Victoria Gillick's (*Gillick* v. *West Norfolk and Wisbech AHA* [1985]) unsuccessful attempt to gain an assurance that her daughters would not be provided with contraceptive advice or treatment without her consent, clearer and more explicit guidelines were produced.

These guidelines made clear that doctors and other health professionals could provide contraceptive advice and treatment to young people provided that certain conditions were met. These are usually referred to as the *'Fraser guidelines'*:

- that the young person understands the advice and has sufficient maturity to understand what is involved (sometimes referred to as *'Gillick Competence'*)
- that the doctor could not persuade the young person to inform his or her parents, nor to allow the doctor to inform them
- that the young person would be very likely to begin or continue having sexual intercourse with or without contraceptive treatment
- that, without advice or treatment, the young person's physical or mental health would suffer
- that it would be in the young person's best interest to give such advice or treatment without parental consent.

Each time a young person consults for treatment an assessment has to be made as to his or her competence to consent to a particular treatment. A young person may have sufficient maturity to consent to one type of treatment, but at the same time not be competent to decide about another type of treatment, e.g. an operation (McHale 1998).

Some barriers for young women in seeking advice on contraception are:

- fear of breaches of confidentiality (very widely held)
- the expectation that they are going to have any request refused
- the belief that they are going to be 'told off'
- rumours that they are going to be 'punished' with some unnecessary procedure, for example:
  - vaginal or pelvic examination
  - cervical smear
- having low self-esteem and low expectations of their needs being met.

Nursing issues

Spend some time thinking about the following:

- gaining accurate knowledge of the legal position
- possessing knowledge of issues specific to young women
- promoting a healthy lifestyle through empowerment
- developing awareness of own prejudices and beliefs
- being aware of the duty of care and confidentiality to the young woman
- having the ability to give appropriate advice and referral criteria
- gaining knowledge of local and national services dedicated to young people.

THE ROLE OF THE SCHOOL NURSE

The school nurse does not have the restraints that teachers have in providing advice and information around contraception and sexual health. The school nurse:

- can give individual advice about contraception to a young woman on a personal basis
- can give general advice and information about contraception that is within the bounds of that school's sex education policy.

Some situations to think about are:

- A very young woman, aged 12 or 13, coming to a clinic or school nurse: did she consent to sex or was coercion used? Are there wider sexual health issues? How old is the boyfriend? What is going on at home? Where is the nearest specialist young peoples' clinic? Is there a child protection issue? What is in the best interest of the young person?
- Addressing the contraceptive needs of those with learning disabilities: does a young woman with a learning disability have the same sexual and reproductive rights and choices as others in the community? Should people who are disabled be encouraged to have sexual relationships? Does educating those with learning disabilities about sex and sexuality encourage them to explore further? Is it the best thing to consider sterilization? Is this a role for the domiciliary family planning service? (Hickerton 1997).
- A 15-year-old wanting an abortion without parental knowledge: what is happening at home? Is there some other family member that can support her? Where is the nearest

specialist young peoples' clinic? Is there a counsellor? Is it possible? (Yes, in exceptional circumstances.)

REFERENCES

BMA, GMCS, HEA, Brook Advisory Centres, FPA and RCGP 1993
    Confidentiality & people under 16
Department of Health 1989 The Children Act. HMSO, London
Hickerton M 1997 Women with special needs and concerns. In: Andrews G (ed)
    Women's sexual health. Baillière Tindall, London, Ch 5
McHale J 1998 Consent to treatment II: children and the mentally ill. In: McHale
    J, Tingle J, Peysner J (eds) Law and nursing. Butterworth Heinemann, Oxford,
    Ch 6

RESOURCES

Brook Advisory Centres (Head Office), 165 Gray's Inn Road, London WC1X
    8UD, UK. Tel.: 020 7713 9000 (information, leaflets and clinics).
Family Planning Association, 2–12 Pentonville Road, London N1 9FP, UK
    (information and leaflets).

4

Young women

This chapter explores some of the issues specific to the health of young women: from the experiences that are common to most, to those that are less frequently encountered. Some of these issues are of social and political importance.

ADOLESCENCE

Adolescence is the transitional period from childhood to adulthood, characterised by experimentation and rapid change (McRae and Rote 1997).

ADOLESCENCE IS A KEY TIME (Forster 1995)

- For learning – especially by exploring new ideas and behaviours.
- For developing values, attitudes and lifestyles.
- For making decisions about health-related activities which will influence future health and well-being.

Some specialist groups for adolescent care are:

- Community drugs team – some areas have set up dedicated drug services for young people (Cohen 1997).
- Child and Adolescent Mental Health Services – providing expert help.
- Young people's clinics – providing dedicated and confidential counselling, advice and help to young people around contraception, sexual health, sexuality and other concerns.
- Bereavement counsellor – the effects of bereavement on young people can be overlooked, with the needs of the adults taking priority.
- Educational psychologist – may be the appropriate specialist for problems at school.

Several opportunities exist for promoting health among adolescents, either planned or opportunistically. They include:

- the school nurse
- the health visitor

Nursing issues

Spend some time thinking about the following:

- knowledge of the many issues particular to young women
- recognize the different rates at which maturity is reached
- understanding the importance of giving full, accurate and unbiased information
- awareness of the social, cultural and religious influences on decision making
- identification of those in particular need of support and care
- awareness of the importance of empowering and enabling adolescents to develop life skills
- how to encourage healthy alliances with local groups
- access to accurate information on local and national resources
- understanding of the issues of consent and confidentiality
- awareness of the importance of the peer group
- understanding that adolescents frequently have difficulty in accessing services.

- the family planning nurse
- the practice nurse
- the outreach worker.

WHAT ARE YOUNG WOMEN WORRIED ABOUT?

Young women are worried about many things, including:

- self-image and esteem
- relationships and communication
- loss and bereavement
- teachers' and parents' expectations (Bowen 1997).

RISK TAKING

Adolescence is the time when people first start trying to find their place in the world. This involves trying out new experiences, which may be risky or even dangerous. It is a time of craving excitement; exciting activities may be dangerous ones. Most experimentation takes place in the presence of others (RCP 1996).

Substance misuse

Youth culture and illegal drug use have been linked for many decades, the particular drug of choice varying according to fashion, trend or availability (Sheehan 1997). Some findings about young people and drug taking (Cohen 1997):

- A third to a half of 15–16-year-olds have used an illegal drug at least once.
- Many young people, in a sample, may have used illegal drugs only once, but over 20% of the total sample were classed as regular users, especially of cannabis.
- 70% have been offered illegal drugs.
- 45% have tried at least one illegal drug at some time in their life.
- There are few differences in drug-using patterns between urban and rural areas, between boys and girls, between black and white, and between different socio-economic groups.

- The use of illicit drugs is most prevalent in the 16–19 and 20–22 age groups.

The reasons for substance misuse are complex and varied, but some factors include (Oliver 1993):

- a means of escape for those who are insecure
- easy availability
- having parents with an alcohol or substance abuse problem
- peer pressure.

Drug use can be difficult to detect, but should be considered in cases of serious, sudden changes in behaviour. The possible effects and risks of drug use will depend on the interaction between (Cohen 1997):

- the drug itself and how it is taken
- the physical and mental health of the drug-taker
- where the drug-taker is, who they are with and what activity they are involved with at the time.

Alcohol

Alcohol is the commonest drug of choice amongst young people. One third of 13–16-year-olds drink alcohol at least once a week. Those in their late teens and early twenties have an alcohol consumption 50% above the adult average, with more heavy drinking and drunkenness than at any other age (Cohen 1997). Alcohol is easily available, provides an escape from insecurity and status may be acquired by drinking large quantities. In later life the adolescent who has abused alcohol may become an alcoholic (Oliver 1993).

Smoking

More girls smoke than boys, with the gender gap starting at an increasingly younger age. It is possible that young women more easily become nicotine dependent. Smoking is also associated with socio-economic status, those in the lower groups smoking more. Poorer women are less likely to give up smoking than men and those with more access to resources. Young women are more likely to use smoking as an appetite suppres-sant to control their weight. Women tend to use smoking as stress relief and part of a coping mechanism (Illman 1997, Woodhouse 1998).

SEX

The average age of first intercourse is 17 years, with 18.7% of young women having had sex for the first time before the age of 16. In a Family Planning Association survey, half of those having first sex before the age of 16 did not use any contraception, while half of young women over the age of 16 used a condom the first time they had sex (FPA 1997). This demonstrates that many young women were ill-prepared for their first sexual experience, either through lack of information and inadequate sex education or through difficulty in accessing appropriate services. It may be reasonable to speculate about how consensual many young women's first sexual experience is.

Key point

Risky behaviour, particularly drug and alcohol abuse increases the risk of accidents, crime, violence, sexual assault, sexually transmitted infections, human immunodeficiency virus (HIV) and unintended pregnancy.

REFERENCES

Bowen C 1997 School survey highlights teenage problem areas. Nursing Times 93 (11)
Cohen J 1997 Young people and drugs. In: Beaumont B (ed) Care of drug users in general practice: a harm minimisation approach. Radcliffe Medical Press, Oxford, Ch 11
FPA 1997 Factsheet No 9 Young people: sexual attitudes and behaviour. Family Planning Association, London
Illman L 1997 Promoting a healthy lifestyle. In: Andrews G (ed) Women's sexual health. Baillière Tindall, London, Ch 1
McRae J, Rote S 1997 Adolescent health: celebrating differences. Primary Health Care 7 (4): 12–14
Oliver R 1993 Psychology and health care. Baillière Tindall, London, Ch 1
RCP 1996 Surviving adolescence. Royal College of Psychiatrists, London
Sheehan A 1997 The teenager and substance abuse. Practice Nursing 8 (10): 28–30
Woodhouse K 1998 Cause for concern: women and smoking. In: Doyal L (ed) Women and health services. Open University Press, Buckingham, Ch 7

FURTHER READING

Forster D A 1995 life-cycle approach to health promotion. In: Pike S, Forster D (eds) Health promotion for all. Churchill Livingstone, Edinburgh, Ch 10

Niven C, Walker A (eds) 1996 Reproductive potential and fertility control. Butterworth-Heinemann, Oxford

Sutherland C 1997 Young people and sex. In: Andrews G (ed) Women's sexual health. Baillière Tindall, London, Ch 4

Woodhouse K 1998 Cause for concern: women and smoking. In: Doyal L (ed) Women and health services. Open University Press, Buckingham, Ch 7

BODY IMAGE

Body image can be described as how an individual interprets his or her body. However the interpretation is influenced by individual and cultural factors (Hendry 1996).

Body image is particularly significant in adolescence and adjusting to a changing body image is especially difficult for adolescents, since there are multiple, simultaneous changes (Grant & Roberts 1998). Adolescents are confronted with the prevailing cultural standards of beauty and attractiveness in relation to evaluating body image. During adolescence greater significance is given to peers as companions, as providers of advice, support and feedback, as models for behaviour and as sources for comparative information; the influence of peers peaks in mid-adolescence (Hendry 1996).

Self-esteem and self-identity are linked to physical appearance, especially in adolescence (Hooton 1998). Adolescence brings weight gain, a change in fat distribution and uneven growth spurts. While some young people are proud of their changing bodies, others are embarrassed by their clumsiness and their budding breasts.

Factors affecting an individual's concept of their body image include the following (Oliver 1993):

- other people's reactions, particularly the opinions and reactions of those whose opinions and judgements are respected
- making comparisons with others
- roles that are adopted
- identification with role models.

DIFFICULTIES WITH BODY IMAGE

- Weight
  - dissatisfaction with weight is a common concern
  - attempts at weight control may progress to an eating disorder (see p. 88).
- Menstruation – some young women are unprepared for this and find it disgusting and frightening.
- Changing body shape – signs of maturing may be unwelcome and frightening (taken to extremes this may be one explanation for anorexia nervosa).
- Acne and other skin problems – it is no longer acceptable to say that it is just a passing phase and to put up with it – there is effective treatment available.
- Breasts – there can be real concerns that breasts are too large, or too small, or of different sizes.
- Body fantasies – misunderstandings about the workings of the body, particularly personal anatomy and physiology, can lead to disabling fantasies (Skrine 1997).
- Dysmorphia – a pathologically abnormal view of body image (e.g. a patently severely anorexic young woman looking in a mirror and seeing a fat image reflected).

Nursing issues

Spend some time thinking about the following:

- knowledge of the physical and psychological changes of puberty
- knowledge of the wide range of 'normal' pubertal changes
- awareness of the emotional fragility of adolescents
- awareness of the importance of peer relationships.

Key points

- Cigarette smoking is frequently believed to aid weight control (Woodhouse 1998).
- A casual and thoughtless remark to a sensitive adolescent about her appearance or behaviour can have far-reaching consequences.
- Body image is not only an issue for adolescents, think of the impact on body image of disease, disability and ageing in all age groups.

REFERENCES

Grant J, Roberts J 1998 Psychological development: sex and sexuality in adolescence. In: Harrison T (ed) Children and sexuality: perspectives in health care. Baillière Tindall, London, Ch 4

Hendry L 1996 Puberty and the psychosocial changes of adolescence. In: Niven C, Walker A (eds) Reproductive potential and fertility control. Butterworth-Heinemann, Oxford, Ch 2

Hooton S 1998 Contemporary cultural influences upon development of sexuality, sexual expression and morality of children living in the UK. In: Harrison T (ed) Children and sexuality: perspectives in health care. Baillière Tindall, London, Ch 2

Oliver R 1993 Psychology and health care. Baillière Tindall, London, Ch 7

Skrine R 1997 Blocks and freedoms in sexual life: A handbook of psychosexual medicine. Radcliffe Medical Press, Oxford, Ch 6

Woodhouse K 1998 Causes for concern: woman and smoking. In: Doyal L (ed) Women and health services. Open University Press, Buckingham, Ch 7

EATING DISORDERS

The two most commonly encountered eating disorders are: anorexia nervosa and bulimia nervosa. Eating disorders are psychological illnesses in which distress is expressed as disordered eating behaviours (Trotter 1997).

The incidence of anorexia nervosa is 1–2 per 1000, with no evidence that the incidence is increasing (Fombonne 1995). It predominantly affects women; only about one in 10 of those with anorexia nervosa are men.

The incidence of bulimia nervosa is at least ten times greater, at 1% of women (Treasure 1989). Because of the more obvious physical effects of anorexia, it is easier to identify someone with anorexia than with bulimia.

Eating disorders are more common in occupations and sports where a low body weight is required. There is a correlation between cultural pressure to be thin and prevalence of eating disorders (Waller 1997)

Eating disorders may be classified according to type, e.g.:

- restrictive in anorexia nervosa
- binge eating/purging in bulimia nervosa.

Mortality in anorexia nervosa is 10%.

Specially trained nurses have a significant role in the treatment and management of those with eating disorders. School nurses are in a key position to identify those at risk of an eating disorder, since pupils may visit her to ask for help because they are concerned about their friend's weight and/or eating habits.

Nursing issues

Spend some time thinking about the following:

- awareness of the characteristics of eating disorders
- alertness to the possibility of an eating disorder
- knowledge of the long-term consequences of eating disorders
- knowledge of management/treatment approaches for different disorders
- understand the pain and fear of the woman that place barriers to treatment
- try to encourage a healthy lifestyle
- provide information about local and national resources
- awareness of referral criteria to a specialist unit

CAUSES

Predisposing factors are:

- family
- personality
- genetic
- adverse events, such as bullying or other abuse of someone who already has low self-esteem.

Precipitating factors are:

- illness, such as a viral illness leading to loss of appetite and weight loss
- weight loss, possibly through effective dieting
- depression
- stress.

Perpetuating factors that arise from the visible weight loss are (Treasure 1989):

- positive social comment ('aren't you lovely and slim, you look just like a model', 'you can't be too thin or too rich', 'whoever heard of an overweight ballet dancer')
- increased family concern
- social isolation
- depression
- decreased sex drive
- painful thoughts blocked, by obsessively concentrating on controlling food-intake.

PRESENTATION

Women with eating disorders either deny that they have a problem or are reluctant to ask for help. A woman may present with another problem, which may itself indicate the possibility of an eating disorder, such as:

- tiredness
- weight loss
- obesity
- menstrual problems
- infertility
- vomiting/constipation/diarrhoea
- dental problems.

ANOREXIA NERVOSA

Peak onset is 16–17 years. It is rare after 35 years.

Diagnostic features

- Refusal to maintain body weight at or above 85% of that expected for age and height
- intense fear of weight gain or becoming fat
- disturbance of perception of body shape, size or weight
- amenorrhoea (the absence of periods for at least three consecutive months).

Fear of being a normal weight drives obsessive restriction of food.

Physical features

Both the physical and psychological features of anorexia nervosa are the consequences of starvation. However, these may not be obvious until BMI is less than 13 (normal range 20–24.9). They include:

- growth of downy hair all over the body
- cardiac complications
- gastrointestinal problems
- kidney failure
- osteoporosis.

Psychological features

Psychological features may include:

- preoccupation with food
- eating rituals
- depression
- poor concentration
- social isolation.

Behavioural features

Some behaviours associated with anorexia are:

- obsessive food rituals, e.g.
  - rigid calorie counting
  - categorization of 'bad' food, by rigid rules of colour or type
  - rigid rules about timing of eating
  - avoidance tactics, suddenly not around at meal times
  - spending hours preparing food and then not eating it
  - obsessive food shopping
- self-induced vomiting
- lying and deceit about food intake
- excessive exercising
- laxative abuse
- diuretic abuse.

Osteoporosis and anorexia nervosa

Adolescents with anorexia are at great risk of developing osteoporosis. The bone loss is related to the duration of illness (Treasure et al 1987).

Peak bone mass is reduced, probably due to a combination of: oestrogen deficiency, malnutrition, and glucocorticoid excess. Moderate exercise can have a beneficial impact on bone density. Excessive exercise, however, can increase the risk of stress fractures. What may start off as 20 minutes a day jogging can develop into 2 to 3 hours of hard running or workout in a gym.

Bone mass remains low despite recovery. Any history of anorexia in adolescence constitutes a risk factor for the premature development of osteoporotic fractures (King 1998).

Treatment and management guidelines (Eating Disorders Association 1998)

- Outcome studies have shown that there is no single form of treatment that works for all people with eating disorders, a range of different types of treatments needs to be available.
- Effective types of treatment include: counselling, psychotherapy, cognitive behaviour therapy, group therapy, family therapy, day hospital programmes, in-patient treatment, dietetic advice, in some instances drugs can be of help in the short term.
- Treatment must address psychological factors associated with eating disorders, such as low self-esteem and anxiety, as well as the eating problem.
- Eating disorders need to be recognized as early as possible before habits are firmly established.
- Services need to be accessible and confidential to encourage people to ask for help.
- In both assessment and treatment the therapist's knowledge and understanding of eating disorders is more important than their specific profession.
- Effective treatment requires the active commitment of the patient. All approaches to treatment should promote autonomy, be flexible, provide choice and enable the development of trust between patient and therapist.
- Care and support may be needed over many years for people with severe or major problems.
- Family and friends need support for themselves, both to help the person with an eating disorder and in order to cope with the impact on their own lives.

BULIMIA NERVOSA

Diagnostic characteristics

Diagnostic characteristics are:

- recurrent episodes of binge eating
- feelings of lack of control over eating during binge eating episode
- regular use of other measures to prevent weight gain
  - self-induced vomiting

- misuse of laxatives, diuretics, etc.
- fasting
- excessive exercising
- binge eating and other activities that occur at least twice a week for a minimum of three months
- persistent over-concern with body shape and weight.

Bulimia is much more common than anorexia, but is easily hidden, with weight frequently being maintained within a reasonable range.

Characteristics of the individual with bulimia nervosa are:

- perfectionist
- dissatisfaction with self and life
- low self-esteem.

Initially, the self-induced vomiting or use of laxatives can give feelings of great release. It may be a way of expressing emotions that are otherwise too difficult to express.

There is a lack of agreement around the significance of the association between bulimia and those who have been abused as children, either physically, sexually or mentally (Sullivan et al 1995).

Some women will continue to binge and purge even when pregnant, resulting in underweight babies.

The long-term consequences of bulimia nervosa are shown in Box 4.1.

Treatment and management

Treatment and education about bulimia nervosa should include:

- education about nutrition
- damage-limitation

Box 4.1 Long-term consequences of bulimia nervosa

- tooth decay due to acid damage of vomit
- irregular menstruation
- damage to gastrointestinal tract e.g. gastric and duodenal ulcers
- constipation after stopping laxatives
- heart and kidney disease
- puffiness of face and fingers, due to fluid retention
- 'hamster' cheeks (enlarged salivary glands from vomiting)
- increased hair growth on face and body
- mineral imbalances.

- cognitive behaviour therapy can be of great help
- counselling for any abuse that may have been experienced.

BINGE-EATING DISORDER

This is disorder of eating that does not meet the diagnostic criteria for anorexia nervosa and bulimia nervosa. It is characterized by chaotic over-eating:

- binge eating
- grazing
- impulsive, unplanned eating
- comfort eating
- eating fast and when not hungry.

The majority of these people are overweight (Waller 1997).

Management and treatment

This will mostly be carried out in primary care, since few will have a sufficiently severe problem that will need to be treated in a specialist centre. Treatment using cognitive behaviour therapy can be effective, incorporating (Waller 1997):

- education
- detailed food and mood diaries
- support and encouragement
- focusing on the eating problem rather than being distracted by other difficulties.

Key point

Referral to a psychiatrist or therapist specializing in eating disorders is essential.

REFERENCES

Eating Disorders Association 1998 Eating disorders – a guide for primary care. Eating Disorders Association, Norwich
Fombonne E 1995 Anorexia nervosa: no evidence of an increase. British Journal of Psychiatry 166: 462–471

King S 1998 A brittle future. Nursing Times 94(1): 23–24

Sullivan P, Bulik C, Carter F, Joyce P 1995 The significance of a history of childhood sexual abuse in bulimia nervosa. British Journal of Psychiatry 167: 679–682

Treasure J 1989 Bulimia nervosa and anorexia nervosa. The Practitioner 233: 1525–1527

Treasure J, Russell FM et al 1987 Reversible bone loss in anorexia. British Medical Journal 295: 474–475

Trotter K 1997 Nutrition and eating disorders. Nutrition in Practice 7. Nursing Times

Waller D 1997 Eating disorders. In: McPherson A, Waller D (eds) Women's health, 4th edn. Oxford University Press, Oxford, Ch 18

FURTHER READING

Palmer RL 1989 Anorexia nervosa: a guide for sufferers and their families, 2nd edn. Penguin, London

Waller D 1997 Eating disorders. In: McPherson A, Waller D (eds) Women's health, 4th edn. Oxford University Press, Oxford, Ch 18

RESOURCES

Eating Disorders Association, First Floor, Wensum House, 103 Prince of Wales Road, Norwich, Norfolk NR1 1DW, UK. Tel.: 01603 621414.

The Mental Health Foundation, 37 Mortimer Street, London W1N 8JU, UK. Leaflets: *All about Bulimia Nervosa*, *All about Anorexia Nervosa*.

MENSTRUATION

Menstruation is the shedding of the endometrium, following the non-fertilization of an ovum. Menarche is the term for the first menstrual period. Menstruation is a normal process, each period indicating the end of one unproductive cycle and the beginning of the next. It starts at puberty, when the internal reproductive organs reach maturity.

The mechanism that initiates puberty is not well understood; however, the levels of gonadotrophin releasing hormone (GnRH) from the hypothalamus increase and so start a chain of events leading to physical maturity (see Box 4.2). It is known that nutrition is important in maintaining normal GnRH function, since underweight women, either deliberately or through disease, do not have periods (though the weight threshold is highly individual) (Chamberlain 1995).

Box 4.2 Physical changes at puberty

- Uterus, uterine tubes and ovaries reach maturity
- Menstrual cycle and ovulation begin
- Breasts develop and enlarge
- Pubic and axillary hair starts to grow
- Increase in rate of growth
- Widening of the pelvis
- Increase in fat deposited in subcutaneous tissue, especially at hips and breasts.

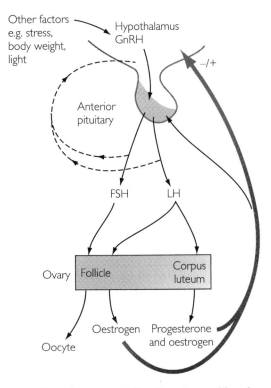

Figure 4.1 Possible pathways controlling the release of female reproductive hormones. GnRH, gonadotrophin-releasing hormone; FSH, follicle-stimulating hormone; LH, luteinizing hormone.

The cycle is determined by the interaction between the hypothalamus, the pituitary gland, the ovaries and the endometrium Figure 4.1 shows the possible pathways involved in the release of female reproductive hormones.

PHASES OF THE MENSTRUAL CYCLE

Figure 4.2 shows a schematic description of menstruation and ovulation. The phases are:

- proliferative or follicular phase
- ovulation
- secretory or luteal phase
- menstruation.

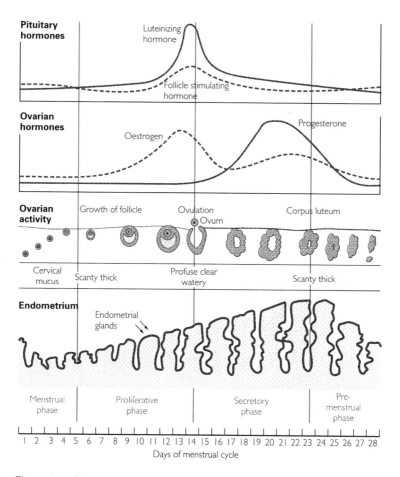

Figure 4.2 Schematic description of menstruation and ovulation. (Modified from Scambler & Scambler 1993, with permission.)

1. *Proliferative phase*
   - follicle-stimulating hormone (FSH) stimulates ovarian follicular growth
   - ovary and maturing follicle produce oestrogen
   - endometrium thickens.
2. *Ovulation*
   - oestrogen reaches peak level
   - luteinizing hormone (LH) surge causes ripened follicle to rupture.
3. *Secretory phase*
   - progesterone continues to cause the endometrium to thicken
   - endometrium is dependent on high levels of oestrogen and progesterone.
4. *Menstruation*
   - non-fertilization leads to degeneration of corpus luteum (the collapsed follicle that produces oestrogen and progesterone)
   - ovarian hormone levels fall, inducing endometrial breakdown (menstruation)
   - low levels of ovarian hormones have a negative feedback effect on the pituitary gland and the hypothalamus, initiating release of FSH and the start of the next cycle.

The proliferative phase can be of variable length. There are normally 12–16 days from ovulation to the onset of menstruation.

Some definitions to do with menstruation are:

- Menarche
  - the first menstrual period
  - usually between 11–15 years
  - average age 12–13 years (in UK).
- Menstrual cycle
  - average is 28 days
  - variations between 21 and 35 days are normal.
- Menstrual period
  - average length 4–5 days
  - 2–8 days can be considered normal
  - average loss 40–50 ml in total
  - loss of upto 80 ml can be normal.
- Menopause is the last menstrual period
  - usually between 45 and 55 years
  - mean being 51 years.

Nursing issues

Spend some time thinking about the following:

- the ability to describe physiology of menstruation
- understanding that menstruation is a natural process
- awareness of the wide range of normal experiences
- awareness of the different cultural attitudes to menstruation (e.g. religious and domestic constraints on Hindu, Muslim and Jewish women while menstruating) (Hickerton 1997)
- awareness of the more common disorders of menstruation
- knowledge of where to access leaflets, etc. about menstruation.
- knowledge of self-help advice for common menstrual disorders (e.g. dysmenorrhoea)
- the ability to 'reassure' and advise concerned parents (usually mothers).

DISORDERS OF MENSTRUATION

Some of the disorders of menstruation are:

- Mittelschmerz – pain following ovulation, may last minutes, hours and occasionally days, probably caused by irritation of the peritoneum by fluid and blood from ruptured follicle.
- Dysmenorrhoea – pain at time of menstruation.
- Amenorrhoea – absence of menstruation.
- Polymenorrhoea – too frequent periods.
- Oligomenorrhoea – infrequent periods.
- Menorrhagia – excessive bleeding.
- Intermenstrual bleeding – bleeding between periods.
- Post-coital bleeding – bleeding after intercourse.

REFERENCES

Chamberlain G (ed) 1995 Gynaecology by ten teachers, 16th edn. Arnold, London
Hickerton M 1997 Women with special needs and concerns. In: Andrews G (ed) Women's sexual health. Baillière Tindall, London, Ch 5
Scambler A, Scambler G 1993 Menstrual disorders. In: Fitzpatrick R, Newman S (eds) The experience of illness. Tavistock/Routledge, London

---

FURTHER READING

Herbert R 1996 Reproduction. In: Hinchliff S, Montague S, Watson R (eds) Physiology for nursing practice, 2nd edn. Baillière Tindall, London, Ch 6.3

TEENAGE PREGNANCY

Teenage pregnancy is associated with increased risk of poor social, economic and health outcomes for both mother and child (Effective Health Care 1997).

WHY IS IT A PROBLEM?

The UK has the highest teenage pregnancy rate among 15 to 19 year olds in western Europe. One-third of all teenage pregnancies are terminated.

INCIDENCE

- Numbers of teenage conceptions have fallen recently, almost certainly in response to greater access to dedicated young people's services.
- Teenage pregnancy rate is considerably higher in deprived and inner-city areas than in more affluent areas (FPA 1997).
- Two-thirds of pregnancies in the more affluent areas are terminated.
- Teenage girls are more likely to have a baby if they
  - have low educational attainment
  - come from families with low socio-economic status and financial hardship
  - had emotional difficulties in childhood or adolescence
  - had a mother who had herself given birth as a teenager.
- In 1994 58.6 in 1000 teenagers became pregnant in England and Wales, down from 69 in 1000 in 1990.
- The Netherlands has the lowest teenage pregnancy rate in western Europe: 10.4 per 1000 aged 15–19 in 1990, almost certainly as a result of a highly effective, compulsory school sex education programme that starts at the beginning of primary education.

THE CONSEQUENCES

Some of the consequences of teenage pregnancy are that

- babies born to teenage mothers are more likely to:
  - be born prematurely
  - weigh less
  - be small for gestational age
- this could be due to socio-economic factors such as low income, poor education and inadequate antenatal care (Davidson 1997)
- young teenagers are more likely to delay seeking advice and care until pregnancy is well advanced (FPA 1997).

PLANNED TEENAGE PREGNANCY

This can be for one or more of the following reasons:

- she may see it as a way of demonstrating her independence
- she may feel she is showing devotion to her boyfriend
- she may be desperate for someone of her own to love
- she may have nothing better to do: no status, no expectations
- she may be worried about infertility, not because she wants a baby now, but because she wants to be sure that she can when she wants to (Sutherland 1997).

UNPLANNED PREGNANCY

Unplanned teenage pregnancy may occur because of:

- lack of information about contraceptive usage and emergency contraception
- embarrassment about discussing contraception with a partner
- unplanned sexual intercourse.

Nursing issues

Spend some time thinking about the following:

- knowledge of issues around teenage pregnancy
- awareness that unplanned may not mean unwanted
- awareness that many teenage pregnancies are very much planned
- knowledge of initiatives to prevent unintended teenage pregnancies
- awareness of the impact of sex education and improved access to contraceptive services
- knowledge of local and national services and resources
- awareness of the importance of providing sensitive, confidential, non-judgemental care.

The *Health of the Nation* (DOH 1992) set the reduction in pregnancies in under 16s, in England, to 50% by the year 2000 as a target:

- 9.5 per 1000 girls aged 13–15 in 1989
- target is no more than 4.8 per 1000
- latest figure of 8.3 in 1994 indicates that target is unlikely to be met.

Counselling a teenager with an unwanted pregnancy may present special difficulties (Davidson 1997). The youngest age group in the lowest socio-economic group are the most vulnerable to inintended pregnancy (FPA 1999).

PREVENTION

Guidelines

Guidelines have been developed by the NHS Centre for Reviews and Dissemination, University of York; *Preventing and reducing the adverse effects of unintended teenage pregnancies*, is a summary of the findings and recommendations (Effective Health Care 1997):

- A good general education is a factor strongly associated with deferring pregnancy.
- School-based sex education can be effective in reducing teenage pregnancy, but it must be linked to access to contraceptive services. The most reliable evidence shows that it does not increase sexual activity or pregnancy rates.
- When used properly, contraceptives are highly cost-effective and can result in significant longer-term savings.
- Increasing the availability of contraceptive clinic services for young people is associated with reduced pregnancy rates.
- Contraceptive services should be based on an assessment of local needs, with accessibility and confidentiality ensured.
- The health and development of teenage mothers and their children has been shown to benefit from programmes promoting access to antenatal care, targeted support by health visitors, social workers or 'lay mothers' and provision of social support, educational opportunities and pre-school education.

REFERENCES

Effective Health Care 1997 Preventing and reducing the adverse affects of unintended teenage pregnancies. Effective Health Care February 3 (2)
Davidson L 1997 Unwanted pregnancy and abortion. In: McPherson A, Waller D (eds) Women's health, 4th edn. Oxford University Press, Oxford, Ch 7
Department of Health 1992 The health of the nation: A strategy for health in England. HMSO, London
FPA 1997 Factsheet No 8 Teenage pregnancy. Family Planning Association, London
FPA 1999 Misconceptions: women's attitudes to planning & preventing pregnancy. FPA, London
Sutherland C 1997 Young people and sex. In: Andrews G (ed) Women's sexual health. Baillière Tindall, London, Ch 4

FURTHER READING

Board of Science and Education 1997 School Sex Education: good practice and policy. British Medical Association, London
Niven C, Walker A (eds) 1996 Reproductive potential and fertility control. Butterworth-Heinemann, Oxford

RESOURCES

NHS Centre for Reviews and Dissemination, University of York, York YO1 5DD, UK. Tel.: 01904 433634 (producer of Effective Health Care).
Brook Advisory Centres (Head Office), 165 Gray's Inn Road, London WC1X 8UD, UK. Tel.: 020 7713 9000.
Family Planning Association, 2–12 Pentonville Road, London N1 9FP, UK. Tel.: 020 7837 5432.

TOXIC SHOCK SYNDROME

Toxic shock syndrome (TSS) is a very rare multi-system disease. It is characterized by rapid onset and is caused by toxins of *Staphylococcus aureus* entering the blood-stream. Recently other pathogens have also been implicated (e.g. *Escherichia coli*) (Rees 1997).

CAUSES

The causes of TSS have been shown to include (Rees 1997):

- half of all cases occur in menstruating women using tampons

- it is associated (in men, non-menstruating women and children) with:
  - hospital-acquired infections
  - surgery
  - boils
  - insect bites
  - burns
  - childbirth
  - contraceptive barriers.

SYMPTOMS

The symptoms are (Gould 1990):

- pyrexia
- skin rash with desquamation (peeling)
- vomiting
- headache
- diarrhoea
- sore throat
- in severe cases dehydration and hypotension rapidly lead to shock.

TSS AND VAGINAL TAMPONS

The exact role of tampons in TSS is uncertain. The role of the absorbency of the tampon has been questioned, with ultra-absorbent tampons probably increasing risk. Some women have recurrences of menstrual TSS even when tampons have not been used (Rees 1997).

It is possible the infection enters the body via the vaginal wall from a tampon which has been left in too long, or which was contaminated before insertion (Steele 1997). Tampon packets now carry a warning about TSS.

Advice on tampon use:

- only use a tampon while menstruating
- wash hands before unwrapping the tampon
- tampons should be changed every 4 to 8 hours
- always check that the last tampon has been removed before inserting a new one
- make sure to remove the last tampon at the end of the period.

Nursing issues

Spend some time thinking about the following:

- knowledge of the rare possibility of TSS
- understanding that it is not necessary to discourage tampon use
- awareness of the importance of promoting good tampon use
- considering advising the use of sanitary pads overnight
- awareness that if TSS is suspected urgent hospital admission and antibiotic treatment is essential.

Key points

- The 'retained' tampon is a common problem:
  - the woman may have forgotten to take out the last tampon
  - she may present with a foul-smelling vaginal discharge.
- The problem is usually resolved by the removal of the tampon.

REFERENCES

Gould G 1990 Women, health and illness. In: Nursing care of women. Prentice Hall, New York, Ch 1
Res 1997 Menstrual problems. In: McPherson A, Waller D (eds) 1997 Women's health. Oxford University Press, Oxford, Ch 10
Steel J 1997 Common gynaecological problems. In: Andrews G (ed) Women's sexual health. Baillière Tindall, London, Ch 16

TURNER'S SYNDROME

Turner's syndrome (TS) is a chromosomal disorder in which one sex chromosome is missing. It may be described as 45XO. The ovaries of fetuses with Turner's syndrome begin to form in the embryo, but undergo a degenerative process by the end of fetal development (Vockrodt & Williams 1994).

Gonadal dygenesis occurs when the ovaries do not develop normally, resulting in the absence of oestrogen production and ova. The ovaries are thin streaks of connective tissue without follicles. TS is estimated to occur in 1 in 2500 live born girls (Kumar et al 1994).

The baby may appear normal at birth. Diagnosis in infants is often suggested by small size, lymphoedema of the hands and feet and excess skin at the nape of the neck (Bartley 1998). Otherwise, the diagnosis may only be suspected later, depending on the variety and severity of the presenting characteristics. This may not be until puberty is expected.

The main characteristics are:

- short stature (less than 150 cm)
- webbed neck
- no secondary sex characteristics
- normal intelligence, but possible learning difficulties (this may be associated with low self-esteem and by parents tending to 'juvenilize' their children) (William 1992)
- cubitus valgus (abnormality of the elbow)
- congenital heart defects, particularly coarctation of the aorta.

Health effects of TS may include.

- cardiovascular disease
- renal disease
- the consequences of long-term oestrogen deficiency.

DIAGNOSIS

Diagnosis is confirmed by chromosomal studies and can usually be carried out pre-puberty since the short stature can easily identify the child. Early diagnosis is important, for the following reasons:

Nursing issues

Spend some time thinking about the following:

- identification of the child with characteristics of TS, may be seen at
  - routine childhood development checks
  - routine immunization
  - at school
- taking parental concerns seriously
- supporting parents and child
- providing information and access to resources
- awareness of health implications
  - cardiovascular defects
  - renal defects
  - consequences of long-term oestrogen deficiency
  - (e.g. osteoporosis, endometrial cancer)
- infertility issues
- effects on the young woman's sexuality
- management options (usually oestrogen, 'opposed' with progestogen to prevent endometrial hyperplasia)

- hormone therapy can be used to stimulate development of the breasts and uterus
- menstruation can sometimes be induced
- issues around fertility can be anticipated.

Turner's syndrome needs to be differentiated from other chromosomal abnormalities, such as the androgen insensitivity syndrome.

Some adults with TS will have been overlooked and will only seek advice with:

- amenorrhoea
- infertility
- difficulties with sexual intercourse may be caused by the absence of oestrogen to stimulate vaginal secretions.

FERTILITY AND TURNER'S SYNDROME

Approximately 5% of women with TS achieve puberty or spontaneously menstruate (Vockrodt & Williams 1994). However, due to the undeveloped uterus and ovaries a spontaneous pregnancy is almost impossible. Assisted conception may be possible with donated oocytes, provided that:

- pelvic scan/hysterosalpingogram demonstrates a uterus capable of sustaining a pregnancy (there is no malformation of the uterus)
- the uterus is receptive to hormonal stimulation, allowing a pregnancy to be sustained and completed.

REFERENCES

Bartley E 1998 Physiological problems. In: Harrison T (ed) Children and sexuality: perspectives in health care. Baillière Tindall, London, Ch 5
Kumar P et al 1994 Molecular biology, genetic disorders and immunology. In: Kumar P, Clark M (eds) Clinical medicine, 3rd edn. Saunders, London, Ch 2
Vockrodt LV, Williams JK 1994 A reproductive option for women with Turner's syndrome. Journal of Pediatric Nursing 9(5): 321–325
Williams J 1992 School-aged children with Turner's syndrome. Journal of Pediatric Nursing 7(1): 14–19

5

Prime time

This chapter explores issues of fertility, fertility control and sexual health. During the prime time in a woman's life these are the most significant health issues. Every woman will be concerned with at least one of these issues at some stage or another.

CONTRACEPTION

Contraception may be defined as the means by which fertility and reproduction are controlled. It is also called family planning or birth control.

WHY IS IT IMPORTANT?

All issues around sexual and reproductive health, and sexuality are of national concern, since they affect the health and well-being of present and future generations (Belfield 1997). In theory, it is Government policy that people should be free to choose where they get their contraception, with GPs providing a service that is complementary to that provided by hospital and community trusts (Executive Letter 1990). The full range of NHS family planning services provided should be appropriate, accessible and comprehensive (NHS Management Executive 1992).

In practice, family planning provision is often seen as a 'soft' target when there are budget cuts, despite a report that suggested that for every £1 spent on family planning services £11 is saved (McGuire & Hughes 1995).

Contraception is much more than fertility control and reasons for attending a family planning clinic include:

- contraception
- pregnancy testing
- unplanned pregnancy
- menstrual problems
- fertility advice
- preconception advice
- infertility
- non-consummation
- sexual difficulties
- sexually transmitted infections (STIs)
- screening (e.g. cervical smears and rubella status)
- relationship problems
- menopause
- breast disorders
- premenstrual syndrome.

ACCESS TO CONTRACEPTIVE SERVICES

Since 1974 all contraceptive services supplied by the NHS are free of charge. NHS contraceptive services can be accessed through the following:

- community family planning clinics
- hospital-based family planning clinics

- dedicated young people's clinics (e.g. Brook Advisory Centres) (age limit varies)
- domiciliary family planning services
- genitourinary medicine (GUM) clinics (e.g. emergency contraception and condoms)
- Accident and Emergency (A&E) departments (e.g. emergency contraception)
- primary healthcare team (PHCT) based in GP surgeries, providing more than 70% of advice and supplies (Belfield 1997)
- 'centres of excellence' (e.g. the Margaret Pyke Centre in London).

There are non-NHS clinics available in most major cities (e.g. Marie Stopes) providing a full range of contraceptive services.

Family planning provision should be:

- comprehensive
- accessible
- efficient and of good quality
- confidential.

A comprehensive service?

Hospital, community and young people's clinics can be expected to offer most, if not all, of the contraceptive methods. However, the service offered in GP practices can vary enormously. One practice may offer a full range of methods, well-trained staff, dedicated session times, with consideration given to other sexual health issues; while another practice may offer the pill and little else. Few practices offer free condoms or pregnancy testing

---

Nursing issues

Spend some time thinking about the following:

- understanding that the woman's personal choice is paramount, and that the nurse's role is to support that choice regardless of any personal views
- understanding the complex and sensitive nature of this area of women's lives
- awareness of the importance of giving full, accurate and objective information
- awareness that a skilled nurse working in this area can make a consultation look very easy, but this level of skill is dependent upon appropriate training
- knowledge of services in area
- providing information and referral as appropriate to specialist services

> **Nursing issues** (continued)
>
> - access to accurate, up-to-date information on the methods available through leaflets, etc
> - awareness of the effect that society, culture, religion, class, family, etc., has on an individual woman's reproductive decisions (Christopher 1996)
> - understanding how contraceptive needs change through a woman's reproductive life
> - demonstrating respect for the woman's decisions and beliefs
> - accurate knowledge of emergency contraception provision and where to access it
> - awareness of the attitudes of society to the reproductive needs and choices of some women, e.g. very young women, older women, those with learning disabilities or who are physically disabled, those with mental health problems, or with complex medical conditions.

GUIDELINES

Family Planning and Contraception in General Practice: Guidance for Nurses (Royal College of Nursing 1996)

CONTRACEPTIVE NEEDS

These can be influenced by (Urwin 1997):

- age
- health
- relationships
- career stage
- financial stability
- decisions about having children.

However, categorizing contraceptive need simplistically and stereotypically by age, parity and social class is denying the factors that influence individual sexual relationships and reproductive choices (Belfield 1997).

CHOICE OF METHOD

Decisions relating to the choice of contraceptive method are influenced by the following (Guillebaud & Hannaford 1998):

- effectiveness
- perceived safety
- recognized contraindications
- acceptability

- ease of use
- availability
- reversibility.

Women's reasons for using and choosing are individual. They include the following (Walsh et al 1996):

- perceptions of self and circumstances
- perceptions and expectations of different methods
- current and foreseeable contraceptive needs, priorities and concerns
- the perceived likelihood of partners agreeing to use of the method
- previous experience of using contraceptive methods and services
- reasons for avoiding pregnancy and degrees of motivation.

Some factors to consider when deciding on a method (Urwin 1997):

- User failure rate as well as method failure rate (the possible failure of the method *per se* or failure of the person to use the method effectively).
- How often the woman needs to think about using the method (e.g. condom before sex, pill every day, injectable contraceptives less frequently).
- Whether the method can be discontinued by the woman (e.g. pill or diaphragm) or whether a health professional needs to remove it (e.g. intrauterine device (IUD) or implants).
- Where it is available.
- Most women will use more than one method of contraception during their reproductive lives.

Efficacy rates of methods

Assume that the method has been fitted correctly (e.g. IUD, intrauterine system (IUS), implant). Assume that the method is being used consistently and correctly.

Information needs

A woman should be given the following information about her chosen method:

- how it works
- how to use it

- efficacy
- advantages
- disadvantages
- possible side-effects.

During the contraceptive consultation:

- Language and culture must be considered when discussing contraception.
- Women seeking contraceptive advice are not 'ill' and do not want their needs medicalized.
- The 'best' method of contraception for an individual woman is that which she has chosen, and which is acceptable to her and her partner.
- There can be much ignorance and misinformation about the workings of the human body and conception.
- Discussion about contraception is a great opportunity for health promotion, both sexual and otherwise.
- It is possible to use more than one method of contraception at a time (e.g. pill and condom, 'double dutch', giving protection against sexually transmitted infections (STIs) at the same time).

Increasing user-effectiveness depends on (Walsh et al 1996):

- ensuring that women know how important it is to use their chosen method correctly and consistently
- teaching women how to use the method correctly
- encouraging disclosure of any problems
- being prepared to discuss women's experiences, perceptions and interpretations of side-effects
- advising on the availability and use of 'back up' methods and of emergency contraception.

CONTRACEPTIVE METHODS

Combined oral contraceptive pill (COC) (British National Formulary 1998)

Stops ovulation – the COC contains hormones similar to those produced by the ovary, and at a level sufficient for the pituitary gland to reduce the production of hormones to stimulate the ovaries for ovulation (Guillebaud 1997).

Advantages:

- reliability
- avoidance of dysmenorrhoea
- less likelihood of iron-deficiency anaemia
- avoidance of premenstrual syndrome
- less benign breast disease
- protection against endometrial and ovarian cancer
- protection against pelvic inflammatory disease (PID).

Disadvantages:

- effectiveness is affected by enzyme-inducing drugs (e.g. those used for tuberculosis and epilepsy)
- increased risk of thromboembolic episodes (e.g. deep vein thrombosis, pulmonary embolism)
- increased risk of arterial disease (myocardial infarction, stroke, peripheral vascular disease) in COC users who smoke, or with other risk factors, and older women
- increases in blood pressure, which usually reverse when COCs are stopped
- possible small increase in risk of breast cancer being diagnosed while using COCs and for up to 10 years after stopping, but the cancers appear to be less advanced and are less likely to have spread beyond the breast (Collaborative Group on Hormonal Factors in Breast Cancer 1996)
- possible increase in risk of cervical cancer in long-term users (Guillebaud & Hannaford 1998).

There are some myths about procedures that need to be carried out before starting the COC. It is not necessary for a woman to undergo a pelvic examination before starting some methods of contraception (e.g. injectables, oral hormonal, implants). Nor is it necessary for young women under the age of 20 to have a cervical smear before starting the oral contraceptive pill.

Progestogen-only pill (POP)

The POP thickens cervical mucus, making a barrier to sperm. It may prevent ovulation in some cycles, and has effects on the endometrium by making it unreceptive to implantation.

Advantages:

- does not interfere with breast-feeding
- particularly useful for those who may have contraindications

to COCs (older women, heavy smokers, history of hypertension, thromboembolism and valvular heart disease).

Disadvantages:

- requires very consistent use
- higher risk of pregnancy among young women
- menstrual irregularities
- possibly same risks of breast cancer as COCs.

Injectable contraceptives (long-acting progestogens)

Injectable contraceptives inhibit ovulation and have some effect on cervical mucus.

Advantages:

- highly effective
- may be used by those who have some contraindications to COCs
- each injection lasts for 12 weeks
- does not interfere with breast-feeding
- reduces risk of endometrial cancer
- may reduce frequency of sickle cell crisis.

Disadvantages:

- if there are side-effects (e.g. depression, facial spots, bloating) they may resolve in time, but may only settle when the method has been discontinued for some time
- possible delay in return to fertility
- irregular bleeding can be erratic and heavy
- amenorrhoea (considered a distinct advantage by many)
- possibly same risks of breast cancer as with COCs.

Implants

These are inserted subcutaneously into upper arm using a fine pre-loaded applicator. They inhibit ovulation, but can also affect cervical mucus and the endometrium.

Advantages:

- highly effective
- long-acting (3 years)

- may be used by those who have some contraindications to COCs
- do not interfere with breast-feeding
- can dramatically reduce menstrual loss
- the rod should not be visible
- rapid return to fertility once the rod has been removed.

Disadvantages:

- rod should be inserted by trained doctor or nurse
- any side-effects are irreversible until rods are removed (e.g. moodiness, depression, facial spots, bloating)
- irregular, sometimes excessive, bleeding in first few months
- contraceptive efficacy reduced by enzyme-inducing drugs
- the rod may be visible (especially on a thin arm).

Intrauterine devices (IUDs)

All IUDs cause a foreign-body reaction in the endometrium, blocking implantation. This reaction is enhanced by copper, which is part of most IUDs, and may inhibit sperm transport, so preventing fertilization. The number of sperm reaching the upper genital tract is fewer in IUD users (Drife 1995).

Advantages:

- highly effective
- long-acting (at least 5 to 8 years)
- does not interfere with breast-feeding
- more effective as emergency contraception than oral form.

Disadvantages:

- if pregnancy occurs miscarriage is more likely
- if pregnancy occurs it is more likely to be ectopic
- small risk of perforation (1 in 1000 insertions) dependent on skill of fitter
- risk of infection, likely to be related to lifestyle, with the highest risk being in first 20 days after insertion and almost certainly related to pre-existing infection
- periods may be heavier and more painful.

Intrauterine system (IUS)

The IUS is a device similar to an IUD, in addition releasing a small daily amount of progestogen.

The endometrium is suppressed, and the device also causes changes to the cervical mucus.

Advantages:

- highly effective
- lasts for 5 years
- does not interfere with breast-feeding
- reduction in menstrual blood loss
- less dysmenorrhoea
- possible reduced risk of clinical pelvic inflammatory disease.

Disadvantages:

- small risk of perforation, dependent on skill of fitter
- risk of infection, highest risk is in first 20 days after insertion and probably related to pre-existing infection
- hormonal side-effects (e.g. mood changes, bloating, facial spots, breast tenderness).

Barrier methods

The barrier is between the male ejaculate and the female genital tract. Barriers can be diaphragms, cervical caps, male and female condoms.

Advantages:

- readily available
- reasonably effective if used properly
- may be considered more 'natural'
- can be used with another method
- does not interfere with breast-feeding
- protection against STIs.

Disadvantages:

- reliant on user-effectiveness
- often perceived as messy, unpleasant or difficult
- spermicide recommended with most barriers.

Natural family planning/fertility awareness (including Persona/ovulation monitor)

These methods allow the woman to recognize and predict ovulation, which occurs 12 to 16 days before the woman's next period.

Advantages:

- can be used to plan pregnancy as well as prevent conception
- no known side-effects
- may be only acceptable method for some couples with particular religious or personal beliefs
- no hormones or devices used
- increased intimacy.

Disadvantages:

- requires commitment from both partners
- efficacy may be only 80 to 98%
- requires careful, consistent observation
- best results from specialist trainers
- may be expensive ('Persona 'is not available on the NHS).

Breast-feeding (lactational amenorrhoea method; LAM)

This gives a reported 98% effectiveness provided:

- the woman is fully breast-feeding (i.e. no supplementary feeds)
- the baby is less than 6 months old
- menstruation has not returned.

Advantages:

- no side-effects
- may be only acceptable method for some couples
- no hormones or devices used.

Disadvantages:

- efficacy is much reduced once supplementary feeding is introduced
- many babies need extra feeding well before 6 months.

Female sterilization

Sterilization means blocking of the uterine tubes to prevent the transport of an ovum to the uterus, by several means:

- clips
- diathermy and cautery
- partial salpingectomy.

Advantages:

- highly effective
- permanent
- can remove the fear of pregnancy, more than with other methods of contraception.

Disadvantages:

- occasional failure (1.5 per 1000)
- not easily reversible
- surgical procedure
- regret, if full counselling has not been carried out, especially in younger women (i.e. under 25 years).

Efficacy of contraceptive methods currently in use (Table 5.1)

Table 5.1   Efficacy of contraceptive methods (Urwin 1997)

Method available	Efficacy	User action
Combined pill	>99%	daily
Progestogen only pill (POP)	99%	daily
Injectables	>99%	infrequent
Implants	>99%	infrequent
Intrauterine device (IUD)	98–99%	infrequent
Intrauterine system (IUS)	>99%	infrequent
Diaphragm	92–96%	before sex
Cervical cap	92–96%	before sex
Male condoms	98%	before sex
Female condoms	95%	before sex
Natural family planning	80–98%	daily
Personal ovulation monitor	94%	daily
Male sterilization (vasectomy)	>99%	never
Female sterilization	>99%	never

EMERGENCY CONTRACEPTION

Emergency contraception is a method of preventing pregnancy that can be used after unprotected sexual intercourse (UPSI), or when there has been a problem with a woman's usual method. Examples of when it might be used include:

- forgetting to take the pill
- condom breaking or coming off during intercourse
- cap not fitted correctly
- lack of communication
- rape or sexual assault
- recent use of drugs likely to affect the fetus (e.g. live vaccines such as rubella or yellow fever).

Emergency contraception works before implantation and so before a pregnancy has been established. There are two main methods: hormonal, through the use of emergency contraceptive pills; or the use of an emergency IUD.

Hormonal methods

Emergency contraceptive pills

- Prevent or delay ovulation.
- May alter the lining of the uterus so that a fertilized ovum is less likely to implant.
- May alter the activity of the muscular wall and the lining of the uterine tubes so that the ovum and sperm are less likely to meet.

Combined oestrogen and progestogen (licensed as PC4) (Yuzpe et al 1982)

- The first two pills are taken within 72 hours of first or only act of UPSI, and the second two pills 12 hours later.
- Failure rate of 1–5%, depending on time in cycle of risk.
- Side-effects of nausea (experienced by <50%) and vomiting (<20%).
- Period should come on time, but may be early or late.

Progestogen-only emergency contraception (POEC) (licensed as Levonelle-2) (Ho & Kwan 1993)

- 0.75 mg of levonorgestrel in each dose.
- First dose within 72 hours of first or only act of UPSI, and the second dose 12 hours later.
- More effective, with a failure rate of 1–2%.
- Causes much less nausea and vomiting.

With both methods it is recommended to start the treatment as soon after the emergency as possible.

Emergency IUD

Copper-releasing IUDs

- Alter the lining of the uterus so that a fertilized ovum does not implant.
- May modify the movement of sperm and so lessen the chance of an ovum being fertilized (Paintin 1998).
- Must be a copper IUD.
- Can be inserted up to 5 days after UPSI, or up to 5 days after the earliest calculated ovulation day in the cycle in question.
- Highly effective (only four documented failures have been reported).
- Risk of concurrent STI must be considered and treated appropriately.

Contraindications (Table 5.2)

Table 5.2 Contraindications of emergency contraception (Kubba & Wilkinson 1998)

Condition	Combined hormonal	Progestogen-only	Copper IUD
Suspected pregnancy	Contraindicated	Contraindicated	Contraindicated
Past history of ectopic pregnancy	Not contraindicated	Not contraindicated	Relative contraindication (can be removed at next period)
Past history of thromboembolism	Relative contraindication	Not contraindicated	Not contraindicated
Migraine at presentation	Contraindicated only if previous history of migraine with aura	Not contraindicated	Not contraindicated

Availability and acceptability of emergency contraception

Emergency contraception is highly effective and very safe. However, there is a general lack of awareness about emergency contraception and how it is obtained, and it should be much more widely available. Currently emergency contraception is available from:

- general practices
- family planning clinics
- youth advisory clinics, e.g. Brook Advisory Centres
- some hospital A & E departments
- some GUM clinics
- some pharmacies are piloting a move to make emergency contraception available directly available without a prescription.

There is no limit to the number of times it can be taken. Fears about breaches of confidentiality can deter some from accessing emergency contraception, especially young women. Some women will not access emergency contraception because of fears of being lectured about their sexual behaviour.

THE FUTURE

There is research being carried out into:

- biodegradable implants
- progestogen-bearing vaginal rings
- oestrogen and progestogen patches
- gels and aerosols
- IUDs ('frameless' devices like the Gynefix, which has copper beads on a thread that is attached to the fundus of the uterus, instead of the current IUD in which copper wire is wound round a plastic frame that fits into the body of the uterus)
- injectables, progestogen-only and combined with oestrogen
- spermicides
- vaccines
- methods of sterilization.

Key point

'The informed user should be the chooser' (Guillebaud 1995).

REFERENCES

Belfield T 1997 FPA contraceptive handbook, 2nd edn. Family Planning Association, London

British National Formulary 1998 Combined oral contraceptives. British Medical Association and Royal Pharmaceutical Society of Great Britain, 7.3.1

Christopher E 1996 Family planning and reproductive decisions. In: Niven CA and Walker A (eds) Reproductive potential and fertility control. Butterworth-Heinemann, Oxford, Ch 7

Collaborative Group on Hormonal Factors in Breast Cancer 1996 Breast cancer and hormonal contraceptives: collaborative reanalysis of individual data on 53 297 women with breast cancer and 100 239 women without breast cancer from 54 epidemiological studies. Lancet 347: 1713–1727

Drife J 1995 Intrauterine contraceptive devices. In: Loudon N, Glasier A, Gebbie A (eds) Handbook of family planning and reproductive health care, 3rd edn. Churchill Livingstone, Edinburgh, Ch 5

Executive Letter EL (90)MB 115 June 1990. Department of Health

Guillebaud J 1995 Advising women on which pill to take. British Medical Journal 311, 28 October, Attachment 1

Guillebaud J 1997 The pill and other forms of hormonal contraception, 5th edn. Oxford University Press, Oxford

Guillebaud J, Hannaford P 1998 Providing high quality contraceptive services in primary care. In: Carter Y, Moss C, Weyman A (eds) RCGP Handbook of sexual health in primary care. RCGP, London

Ho PC, Kwan MSW (1993) A prospective randomized comparison of levonorgestrel with the Yuzpe regimen in post-coital contraception. Human Reproduction 8: 389–392

Kubba A, Wilkinson C 1998 Recommendations for clinical practice: emergency contraception. Faculty of Family Planning and Reproductive Health Care of the Royal College of Obstetricians and Gynaecologists, London

McGire A, Hughes D 1995 The economics of family planning services. Family Planning Association, London

NHS Management Executive 1992 Guidelines for reviewing family planning services: guidance for regions. Department of Health, London

Paintin D 1998 Twenty questions about emergency contraception – answered. Birth Control Trust, London

RCN 1996 Family planning and contraception in general practice: guidance for nurses. Issues in nursing and health 41. Royal College of Nursing, London

Urwin J 1997 Current issues in contraception. Primary Health Care 7(8): 31–36

Walsh J, Lythgoe H, Peckham S 1996 Contraceptive choices: supporting effective use of methods. Family Planning Association, London

Yuzpe AA, Smith RP, Rademaker AW (1982) A multicenter clinical investigation employing ethinyloestradiol combined with dl-norgestrel as a postcoital contraceptive agent. Fertility and Sterility 37: 508–513

FURTHER READING

Andrews G (ed) 1997 Women's sexual health. Baillière Tindall, London

Belfield T 1997 FPA Contraceptive handbook, 2nd edn. Family Planning Association, London

Clubb E, Knight J 1997 Fertility. David & Charles, Newton Abbot

Everett S 1998 Handbook of contraception and family planning. Baillière Tindall, London

Guillebaud J 1999 Contraception: your questions answered, 3rd edn. Churchill Livingstone, London

Guillebaud J 1997 Contraception. In: McPherson A, Waller D (eds) Women's health, 4th edn. Oxford University Press, Oxford, Ch 6

Loudon N, Glasier A, Gebbie A (eds) 1995 Handbook of family planning and reproductive health care, 3rd edn. Churchill Livingstone, Edinburgh

---

RESOURCES

Brook Advisory Centres (Head Office), 165 Gray's Inn Road, London WC1X 8UD, UK. Tel.: 020 7713 9000
Family Planning Association, 2–12 Pentonville Road, London N1 9FP, UK. Tel.: 020 7837 5432
Fertility UK, Clitheroe House, 1 Blythe Mews, London W14 0NW, UK. Tel.: 020 7371 1341

PRECONCEPTION CARE

Preconception care is the advice given to a couple about health issues that (Defriez 1997):

- optimize the health of the woman and her partner before conceiving
- affect the chance of conception
- decrease the chance of congenital abnormalities
- decrease the risks of recurrent miscarriage.

The aims are (Illman 1997):

- to give a baby the best possible start in life by minimizing risks associated with lifestyle, heredity, medical history and maternal age
- to promote the health of the mother.

Nursing issues

Spend some time thinking about the following:

- awareness that planning a pregnancy and making changes are best done before conception occurs
- preparedness to carry out opportunistic health promotion: it is never too late to make some changes, even when pregnant
- how to demonstrate sensitivity and understanding concerning the complexities in some women's lives that limit the choices they can make
- understanding of the need for women to have antenatal care
- knowledge of antenatal screening issues
- awareness of the need of some couples to be referred for specialist genetic counselling
- awareness that women with pre-existing conditions (e.g. diabetes, epilepsy, cardiovascular or renal disease) need specialist care.

WEIGHT

Underweight women are less likely to conceive, because of amenorrhoea or infrequent periods and more likely to have underweight babies. Overweight women or obese women have reduced fertility and more problems in pregnancy. Women should not 'diet' during pregnancy, but aim to lose weight before conceiving.

DIET

Diet should be healthy, well-balanced and rich in folic acid, to reduce the possibility of neural tube defects (spina bifida). The Department of Health (DOH 1992) recommends that all women take a supplement of folic acid starting before conception and continuing until they are 12 weeks pregnant:

- to prevent first-time occurrence of spina bifida, 0.4 mg daily
- to prevent recurrence (in women who have already had one baby with spina bifida), 5 mg daily
- women with epilepsy will need the higher supplement and specialist advice before planning a pregnancy (many of the anticonvulsants produce a higher incidence of neural tube defect and other abnormalities) (Whittle & Hanretty 1986)

Women should avoid, while pregnant, foods that may be contaminated with *Listeria* which can cause:

- miscarriage
- still-birth
- severe illness in the newborn baby.

Women should also avoid foods that may be infected with *Salmonella*. Foods to avoid are:

- soft cheeses
- pâtés
- raw or undercooked eggs
- poultry
- cook–chill foods.

Women should avoid foods rich in vitamin A, as high doses can affect fetal development. Foods to avoid are liver and liver products.

ALCOHOL

It appears safe for a pregnant woman to drink 1 to 2 units once or twice a week. Excessive alcohol:

- may be particularly damaging in early pregnancy
- can reduce a man's sperm count
- may contribute to miscarriage
- is associated with low birth-weight and congenital abnormalities.

Alcohol dependency can cause fetal alcohol syndrome (FAS).

SMOKING

Smoking in men reduces testosterone levels and increases the numbers of abnormal sperm.

Smoking in women:

- increases incidence of ectopic pregnancy and miscarriage
- produces more low-birth-weight babies
- increases risk of atopic disease (e.g. asthma, eczema)
- is associated with sudden infant death syndrome (SIDS), though this is mainly due to the smoky atmosphere resulting from parental smoking.

DRUGS

Some drugs affect fetal development. Advice should always be sought before taking any drugs or treatment, including those which are:

- prescribed
- over-the-counter (OTC)
- recreational.

Women who are dependent drug-users will need specialist support throughout their pregnancy.

RUBELLA

Rubella infection in the first 10 weeks of pregnancy causes congenital rubella syndrome in 90% of those infected. Women should always be checked for the presence of rubella antibodies regardless of rubella infection in past. Immunization in childhood or adolescence is no guarantee of a protective antibody response level.

GENETIC TESTING

If a genetic disorder is known or suspected, referral should be made to a specialist genetics centre, where the couple can receive:

- risk assessment and genetic counselling
- diagnostic opinion
- family studies
- prenatal diagnosis
- follow-up counselling and support.

Key points

- Up to 50% of pregnancies may be unplanned, therefore preconception advice should be given opportunistically.
- Low birth-weight is a major cause of perinatal mortality.
- Low birth-weight is associated with maternal health and lifestyle and lower socio-economic group.

REFERENCES

Defriez M 1997 Preconceptional care and advice. Primary Health Care 7 (2): 31–38
Department of Health 1992 Folic acid and the prevention of neural tube defects. Report from an Expert Advisory Group. HMSO, London
Illman L 1997 Promoting a healthy lifestyle. In: Andrews G (ed) Women's sexual health. Baillière Tindall, London, Ch 2
Whittle M, Hanretty K 1986 Prescribing in pregnancy. British Medical Journal, 293: 1485–1488

PREMENSTRUAL SYNDROME

Premenstrual syndrome is a combination of affective (emotional) and somatic (physical) symptoms that begin around the luteal phase and usually diminish after menstruation begins (Edge & Miller 1994).

There is no agreed definition of premenstrual syndrome (PMS); however, there are certain characteristics to the collection of symptoms.

The symptoms:

- are cyclical
- become apparent after ovulation
- are relieved by the onset of menstruation.

The symptoms can be:

- physical
- psychological
- behavioural.

The severity of the symptoms can be from mild to debilitating. The syndrome was first described by Frank in 1931, and for many years it was called premenstrual tension (PMT). It has been questioned whether the term 'syndrome' should be used at all, since syndrome refers to a group of symptoms that occur together and characterize an abnormal condition. Many of the core symptoms of PMS are so widespread among the majority of women as to be almost 'normal' (Richardson 1995).

PMS is associated with ovarian activity since the symptoms appear after ovulation. The condition does not occur:

- before puberty
- during pregnancy
- after the menopause.

It can continue after hysterectomy if the ovaries have been preserved (Magos et al 1986).

INCIDENCE

Mild physiological symptoms are present in 95% of women of reproductive age. Five percent of women suffer severe and disruptive premenstrual symptoms (O'Brien 1993). Any woman can have PMS. There is no consistent relationship between women's personalities and PMS. However, there appear to be links between PMS and general psychological health. Women tend to experience PMS as more of a problem during times of stress, and some women may be more vulnerable than others to hormonal fluctuations (Gardner & Sanders 1997).

CAUSES

There have been many theories as to the cause of PMS, most theories being proved and then disproved. Not all theories have been rigorously researched, however, relying more on anecdotal evidence. Some theories of possible causes of PMS include:

- progesterone deficiency
- oestrogen/progesterone imbalance
- nutritional deficiency
- prostaglandin imbalance
- raised prolactin levels
- fluid and electrolyte imbalance
- hypoglycaemia
- serotonin imbalance.

Causes are almost certainly multi-factorial. Current consensus is that PMS is caused by an abnormal neurotransmitter response to normal ovarian function (O'Brien 1993).

Current research focuses on three areas:

- hormone imbalance
- nutritional deficiency
- neurotransmitter abnormality.

As long ago as 1979 a review of the research literature produced evidence for and against every theory and concluded that no single treatment was more effective than any other (BMJ 1979).

SYMPTOMS

As many as 150 symptoms are attributed to PMS. Those most commonly accepted are:

- Physical symptoms:
  - breast pain
  - fluid retention
  - headache
  - abdominal bloating
  - dizziness/faintness
  - constipation or diarrhoea
  - changes in appetite

- skin eruptions
- muscle stiffness.
- Psychological symptoms:
  - depression
  - aggression/tension
  - irritability
  - clumsiness
  - change in sex drive
  - fatigue.
- Behavioural symptoms:
  - lack of concentration
  - decreased work performance
  - absenteeism.

DIAGNOSIS

Diagnosis is made through taking a thorough history. If there is any doubt about the diagnosis, charting a symptom diary for 3 months will clarify the situation. Chart symptoms to identify their range, frequency, duration and severity. Also chart any other factors that may contribute to the symptoms. A menstrual diary can help to assess the occurrence of symptoms in relation to the menstrual cycle.

No one blood test is of any diagnostic value; for example, progesterone is a pulsatile hormone, therefore levels will fluctuate from day to day.

TREATMENT

Treatment should be targeted at the woman's worst symptoms. Simpler interventions should be tried first where there are more

---

Nursing issues

Spend some time thinking about the following:

- listening and being sympathetic to the woman
- believing the woman's symptoms
- trying to find out and understand the stresses and difficulties in her life
- finding out what has prompted her to seek help now
- encouraging a healthy lifestyle
- awareness of recognized self-help therapies
- the ability to provide access to information and other resources
- being prepared to act as the woman's advocate.

psychological symptoms. There can be a very high placebo response to any intervention: 94% was cited by Magos et al in 1986, although a rate of 50% is generally accepted. This is probably due to the therapeutic effect of acknowledging and discussing the woman's individual situation. Treatments include lifestyle, diet and stress reduction, non-hormonal treatments and hormonal treatments.

Lifestyle, diet and stress reduction

- Rest, exercise and stress reduction appear to increase natural endorphins and decrease symptoms.
- Psychotherapy, counselling, meditation or yoga can help some women.
- Fatigue and stress exaggerate discomfort, therefore maintaining a healthy diet, increasing intake of complex carbohydrates, fruit and vegetables, limiting intake of salt, caffeine, saturated fat, sugary foods and alcohol may help.
- Eating frequent meals prevents low blood sugar, implicated in headaches and irritability.

Non-hormonal treatments

- Prostaglandin inhibitors (e.g. mefenamic acid, naproxen) may reduce headache and irritability.
- Gamma linolenic acid (in evening primrose oil and starflower oil) can help breast pain.
- Diuretics may help proven fluid retention and bloating.
- Pyridoxine (vitamin B_6) has been much used with little evidence that it has any beneficial effect (long-term use with higher doses may lead to peripheral neuropathy).
- Other mineral and vitamin supplements are promoted, again with little evidence as to mode of action or beneficial effect, and include magnesium, zinc and vitamin B.
- Many women report benefits from alternative therapies including acupuncture, homeopathy, aromatherapy, reflexology and herbal medicine.
- Antidepressants, particularly serotonin re-uptake inhibitors (SSRIs), can help some women (O'Brien 1993).

Hormonal treatments

- Combined oral contraceptive pill prevents ovulation – and therefore the onset of the luteal phase – and is effective for some women, especially if taken tricyclically (continuously for three packets without a break).
- Progesterone vaginal pessary (following the theory of progesterone deficiency) 200–400 mg daily from 14 days before anticipated period until onset of menstruation (Magill 1995).
- Oestrogen suppresses ovulation. When given initially as 100 μg oestradiol subcutaneous implant there are definite benefits (Magos et al 1986). High dose oestrogen patches are also helpful (Andrews 1997). Oestrogen needs to be 'opposed' with progestogen, for around 12 days each cycle, to prevent endometrial hyperplasia (see p. 176).
- Danazol, a synthetic hormone that suppresses ovulation, although the androgenic side-effects are unacceptable to many.
- Gonadotrophin releasing hormone (GnRH) analogues inhibit ovarian function, can be given by monthly implant (goserelin) or daily nasal spray (buserelin); long-term use is restricted due to risks associated with oestrogen deficiency, especially osteoporosis (see p. 192).

Other remedies

Surgery is a rare and extreme resort. Hysterectomy and bilateral oophorectomy may be considered if:

- the woman is in her 40s with very severe symptoms
- the woman was due to have a hysterectomy for menorrhagia, when the ovaries would usually be conserved.

Key points

- Society has come to expect women to be 'out of control' premenstrually.
- Attributing premenstrual feelings to uncontrollable forces may be a way of avoiding solving situational and personal problems (Chamberlain 1995).

REFERENCES

Andrews G 1997 Can HRT relieve premenstrual syndrome symptoms? Nurse Prescriber, Community Nurse, October 1997: 33–34

BMJ 1979 Premenstrual tension syndrome. British Medical Journal, 286: 212

Chamberlain G (ed) 1995 Gynaecology by ten teachers, 16th edn. Arnold, London, Ch 11

Edge V, Miller M (eds) 1994 Women's health care. Mosby, St. Louis, Ch 4

Frank RT 1931 The hormonal causes of premenstrual tension. Archives of Neurology and Psychiatry 26: 1053–1057

Gardner K, Sanders D 1997 Premenstrual syndrome. In: McPherson A, Waller D (eds) Women's Health, 4th edn. Oxford University Press, Oxford, Ch 9

Magill PJ 1995 Investigation of the efficacy of progesterone pessaries in the relief of symptoms of premenstrual syndrome. British Journal of General Practice 45: 589–593

Magos AL, Brincat M, Studd JWW 1986 Treatment of the premenstrual syndrome by subcutaneous oestradiol implants and cyclical oral norethisterone: placebo controlled study. British Medical Journal 292: 1629–1633

O'Brien PMS 1993 Helping women with premenstrual syndrome. British Medical Journal 307: 1471–1475

Richardson JTE 1995 The premenstrual syndrome: a brief history. Social Science and Medicine 41(6): 761–767

FURTHER READING

Andrews G 1997 Premenstrual syndrome. In: Andrews G (ed) Women's sexual health. Baillière Tindall, London, Ch 13

Evennett K 1995 Coping successfully with PMS. Sheldon, London

Shreeve C 1992 Premenstrual syndrome. Thorsons, London

RESOURCES

National Association of Premenstrual Syndrome (NAPS), PO Box 72, Sevenoaks, Kent TN13 1XQ, UK. Tel.: 01732 741709.

The Premenstrual Society (PREMSOC), PO Box 429, Addlestone, Surrey KT15 1DZ, UK. Tel.: 01932 872560.

Women's Health, 52 Featherstone Street, London EC1Y 8RT, UK. Tel.: 020 7251 6580.

PROBLEMS RELATED TO CHILDBEARING

Some women experience difficulty in becoming pregnant or in sustaining the pregnancy. This may be due to disease or other abnormality of the genital tract or other pelvic organs.

Nursing issues

Spend some time thinking about the following:

- awareness of some of the problems around conception and sustaining a pregnancy
- understanding of the distress, anxiety and trauma experienced by the woman, and her partner
- appreciating the issues around future fertility for that woman
- awareness of some of the management options
- knowledge of local and national resources, and self-help groups.

Conditions that prevent conception or a pregnancy continuing to full term are as follows.

CERVICAL STENOSIS

This condition almost always occurs as a result of cervical surgery, usually a cone biopsy. It can lead to complete occlusion of the cervical canal, so preventing conception.

INCOMPETENT CERVIX

Incompetent cervix is one of the most common causes of late spontaneous abortion. Diagnosis is usually made after a miscarriage, usually mid-trimester. It may be caused by the cervix tearing during a previous normal labour or during forceps delivery. It may follow on from excessive dilatation of the cervix during a surgical procedure, usually a termination of pregnancy. Management is usually by inserting a pursestring suture (Shirodkar) around the cervix early in the second trimester of pregnancy that will hold the cervix closed as the pregnancy progresses. The suture is removed at 38 weeks or at the onset of labour; this procedure is successful for many (Sweet 1988).

FIBROIDS (see p. 294)

These are balls of muscle arising from the myometrium or uterine muscle. They are not usually associated with infertility, but may cause difficulties if large enough to distort the uterine cavity or when their situation occludes access of sperm to the uterine tubes. They rarely cause a miscarriage, but may do so if large and protruding into the uterine cavity. A myomectomy, the surgical removal of a fibroid, may be carried out for infertility or recurrent miscarriage if no other cause can be found.

VAGINAL ABNORMALITIES

There may be an absent or incomplete vagina, or one that is unconnected to the uterus. This may be the result of a failure of embryological development. It can be possible for these abnormalities to be corrected by plastic surgery.

UTERINE ABNORMALITIES

These are caused by incomplete fusion of Mullerian ducts during fetal development. The abnormality may be one or more of the following:

- double uterus, double cervix and double vagina
- double uterus and one cervix
- uterus with a septum
- small deformed uterus (one Mullerian duct has not developed at all).

Uterine abnormalities may cause habitual abortion or premature labour, while a double vagina or septum may cause haemorrhage during labour. Any reconstructive surgery may be at risk of rupture during labour.

ECTOPIC PREGNANCY

A fertilized ovum usually implants in the endometrium. If implantation is sited anywhere else this is an ectopic pregnancy. Fertilization usually takes place in the uterine tubes, in the ampulla, from where the fertilized ovum is wafted down into the uterus. The differential diagnosis of ectopic pregnancy is shown in Box 5.1.

Ninety per cent of ectopic pregnancies are sited in the uterine tubes (other sites are ovary, cervix and abdominal cavity). If the tube ruptures as the pregnancy advances the bleeding can be life-threatening. If the tube has not ruptured, an attempt is made to remove the pregnancy and conserve the tube, using laparoscopic techniques, though there is a risk of a further ectopic pregnancy. If the tube ruptures there is usually profuse bleeding and a

Box 5.1 Differential diagnosis of ectopic pregnancy
Ectopic pregnancy may be confused with
• pelvic inflammatory disease • miscarriage • rupture of an ovarian cyst • torsion of an ovarian cyst • appendicitis.

salpingectomy (removal of uterine tube) needs to be carried out urgently.

Ectopic pregnancy is most likely to occur when there has previously been pelvic infection or tubal surgery. It has been suggested that the progestogen-only pill (POP) may increase the risk by affecting the motility of the uterine tubes, slowing down the rate at which the fertilized egg is transported to the uterus (Fraser 1995), although this has not been confirmed.

ENDOMETRIOSIS (see p. 287)

Mild endometriosis does not appear to affect fertility, and may be only an incidental finding. However, moderate and severe disease can cause adhesions around the uterine tubes, and ovarian cysts. Laser surgery can remove the adhesions and restore the anatomy and possible fertility. Some women will need assisted conception techniques.

Women who experience dyspareunia (pain with sex) are likely to have sexual intercourse infrequently, and so reduce the opportunities for conceiving.

REFERENCES

Fraser I 1995 Progestogen-only contraception. In: Loudon N, Glasier A, Gebbie A (eds) Handbook of family planning and reproductive health care, 3rd edn. Churchill Livingstone, Edinburgh, Ch 4
Sweet B (ed) 1988 Operative procedures in obstetrics. In: Mayes' midwifery, 11th edn. Baillière Tindall, London, Ch 44

FURTHER READING

Moulder C 1998 Understanding pregnancy loss. Macmillan, Basingstoke

RESOURCES

The Miscarriage Association, PO Box 24, Ossett, West Yorkshire WF5 9XG, UK.
Stillbirth and Neonatal Death Society (SANDS), 28 Portland Place, London
    W1N 3DE, UK. Tel.: 020 7436 5881.

INFERTILITY

Infertility is generally defined as the involuntary failure to
conceive within 12 months of commencing unprotected intercourse (Joels & Wardle 1994). Others suggest that the timescale is
two years failure to conceive.

INCIDENCE

Ninety per cent of couples will conceive within 12 months of
starting to try, where the female partner is aged under 35. Most
other fertile couples will conceive during the following 12 months
(Lockwood 1997).
    Using a definition of two years without achieving a pregnancy:

- 1 in 8 couples will seek help to have their first child
- half may conceive spontaneously or with medical help
- 8% do not achieve desired family size
- 4% never experience a pregnancy (Bennett & Templeton
  1995).

There is a natural decline in the fertility of women after the age of
35. Many couples are subfertile rather than infertile. There are
both male and female factors in infertility.
    Infertility can be:

- primary, where the woman has never been pregnant
- secondary, where there have been one or more previous
  pregnancies, whatever the outcome.

Overall, one in six couples will seek specialist help at some time
because of infertility. There has been no increase in the prevalence
of infertility in the past 10 years; the much increased demand for
specialist services is probably due to greater public awareness
(Joels & Wardle 1994).

For conception to occur there are a number of essential elements (Chamberlain 1995):

- ovulation
- patent, functional uterine tubes
- normal cervix and uterus
- intercourse at appropriate time in ovarian cycle
- sperm of an adequate quality and quantity.

The main causes of infertility are:

- sperm dysfunction and other male factors such as failure of ejaculation (>24%)
- ovulation disorder (21%)
- tubal disorder (14%)
- endometriosis (6%)
- cervical mucus hostility (2%)
- uterine abnormalities (2%)
- unexplained (28%).

Ten to 15% of couples will have more than one abnormality.

EFFECTS OF INFERTILITY

Chamberlain (1995) describes the failure to conceive as a stressful cycle of continual hope and disappointment. Individuals will experience the following:

- failure (not a 'real' woman or man)
- guilt or shame (e.g. for having had a sexually transmitted infection or an abortion)
- selfish (for having delayed trying to conceive or for wanting another child)
- anger – with self or partner, or both
- anger with society, for example, for allowing environmental factors to affect sperm quality or for inequalities in access to treatments
- anger with friends, colleagues, family, etc., for their expectations and beliefs
- low self-esteem (not worthy enough)
- isolation (difficulty in mixing with friends with babies)
- detrimental effect on sexual and other relationships
- anxiety and depression

- financial cost (assisted conception techniques are very expensive)
- lack of understanding for the woman who does not have a partner or who is in a lesbian relationship and who wants a child.

Each couple should have their particular set of circumstances assessed on an individual basis. Some basic misunderstandings may effect their ability to conceive. For example:

- Never assume that a couple consulting about a failure to conceive are having regular, penetrative vaginal intercourse (some couples have a problem with non-consummation; some couples are living apart, even in other countries; partner may be in prison).
- Never assume that the couple have the knowledge to identify their 'fertile period'.
- A prolonged period of abstinence will not 'strengthen' poor sperm (Lockwood 1997).

INVESTIGATIONS

All baseline investigations for infertility can be carried out in the primary care setting. The initial history, examination and investigation should be directed at confirming:

- ovulation
- adequate and normal sperm production
- tubal patency
- normal intercourse (Blunt & Walker 1997).

A full history should include:

- age (of both partners)
- duration of the problem
- previous pregnancies and their outcome
- frequency of intercourse
- any pain or difficulty with intercourse
- any problems with menstruation
- previous infections, e.g. pelvic inflammatory disease or a sexually transmitted infection (STI), especially *Chlamydia* (see p. 161)
- medical disorder

- contraceptive history
- previous pelvic surgery
- occupational and domestic circumstances.

Both partners must be investigated.

LIFESTYLE FACTORS AFFECTING FERTILITY (see p. 126)

- Weight:
  - obesity may be associated with polycystic ovary syndrome (PCOS) (see p. 318)
  - severely underweight women are likely to have irregular or absent periods.
- Smoking, alcohol and drugs can affect sperm production in the male and fetal development in the female.
- Occupation: there may be hazards in the work environment.
- Psychological factors (e.g. stress and anxiety).

NB, discussing fertility problems should be taken as an opportunity to inform the woman about the full range of preconception issues.

EXAMINATION

- General examination – for signs of endocrine disorder (e.g. hirsutism in PCOS).
- Abdominal examination – for signs of abdominal or pelvic surgery, or tenderness.
- Bimanual pelvic examination
  - for signs of structural abnormality
  - tenderness or reduced mobility of pelvic structures
  - adnexal masses (e.g. ovarian cyst, salpingitis, fibroid, or abcess).

Every woman must have her rubella status confirmed.

Apart from sperm dysfunction, ovulation disorders are the commonest cause of infertility. The main causes of anovulation (failure to ovulate) are as follows:

- polycystic ovary syndrome
- hypothalamic dysfunction

  – drugs
  – anorexia
  – obsessive exercising
- pituitary disease or dysfunction
- thyroid dysfunction
- adrenal dysfunction
- ovarian dysfunction or failure
- diabetes
- radiotherapy/chemotherapy.

Tests to confirm ovulation involve investigation of the hypothalamic–pituitary–ovarian axis. In the follicular phase this is to investigate levels of follicle-stimulating hormone (FSH) and luteinizing hormone. In the luteal phase it is to investigate levels of progesterone (day 21 of 28-day cycle).

If the periods are scanty, infrequent or absent, or the woman is hirsute the following hormones will be checked:

- testosterone
- prolactin
- thyroid-stimulating hormone.

Any further tests will be carried out by a specialist unit. These will include:

- serial ultrasound scanning to track the development of a dominant follicle
- tests of tubal patency
  – laparoscopy (to identify adhesions, endometriosis, fibroids, or any abnormality of the external structure of uterus, uterine tubes or ovaries)
  – hysterosalpingogram (radio-opaque dye is injected into the uterus, through the cervix, and then passes through the uterine tubes, demonstrating any obstruction or abnormality of the uterine cavity or tubes)
- postcoital testing to demonstrate receptivity of cervical mucus and ability of sperm to reach and survive mucus.

TREATMENT (see p. 147 and Box 5.2)

- Treatment will depend on the probable cause.
- Accurate diagnosis of the problem is essential.
- In many couples there is more than one factor.

Box 5.2	Some conditions and their treatment/management options
Disorders of ovulation Premature ovarian failure Blocked tubes Abnormal or absent uterus Sperm of poor quality/quantity	Ovulation induction with drugs Ovum donation Tubal surgery and/or assisted conception Surrogacy Artificial insemination by partner or donor or assisted conception

Disorders of ovulation and unexplained infertility have the best chance of responding to relatively simple procedures (Lockwood 1997).

Ovulation induction can be carried out in primary care, only when the precise fertility problem has been diagnosed. However, some people with a fertility problem should always be referred to a specialist centre (Power 1997):

- women over 35 years with 6–12 months of subfertility
- women with more than 1 year of subfertility
- women with ovarian failure who have a raised FSH
- failure to respond to clomiphene (used for ovulation induction)
- possible tubal or pelvic disease
- abnormal semen analysis
- negative post-coital test.

COUNSELLING

Counselling has a role in supporting people who are infertile at any stage, and is required in some assisted conception techniques. Counselling should be considered a normal step in the psychological process through infertility. It offers the following (Mack & Tucker 1996):

- information about investigations and treatment options
- a safe space to express anger, frustration, guilt and fear
- help to deal with the initial feelings of loss, disappointment and failure
- support for communication between the couple
- understanding of the implications of donated gametes (egg, sperm or embryo)

- help with making the decision to start or continue treatment
- support for the decision to stop treatment without a pregnancy
- discussion and exploration of expectations
- counselling for childlessness.

Nursing issues

Spend some time thinking about the following:

- awareness of the incidence of infertility
- knowledge of some of the causes, investigations and treatments
- awareness of some of the psychological effects on the woman, her partner and other relationships
- understanding the embarrassment and stress that can be caused by the whole process of investigation and treatment
- awareness of the importance of support, through counselling or support groups, or both
- understanding the need for a non-judgemental approach to each woman and her needs
- knowledge of access to specialist centres locally and nationally, and contrasting policies that may apply in neighbouring areas
- awareness of the Human Fertilisation and Embryology Authority (HFEA), including its role, Code of Practice and patient leaflets and guides (see p. 146)
- understanding of the role of the specialist fertility nurse, and means of access.

Key points

- Questions asked at this time are intensely personal and intimate, it being necessary to reveal details of past and present sexual behaviours and practices. Some of this information may not be known by the partner.
- Judgements may be made about the suitability or worthiness of one woman over another in the lottery for infertility treatment.

REFERENCES

Bennett S, Templeton A 1995 The epidemiology of infertility. In: Meerabeau L and Denton J (eds) Infertility: nursing and caring. Scutari Press, London, Ch 3

Blunt S, Walker D 1997 Infertility and pregnancy loss. In: Luesley DM (ed) Common conditions in gynaecology. Chapman & Hall, London, Ch 7

Chamberlain G (ed) 1995 Sexual and reproductive health. In: Gynaecology by ten teachers, 16th edn. Arnold, London, Ch 11

Joels LA, Wardle PG 1994 Causes and treatment of infertility. British Journal of Midwifery, Infertility Supplement 2 (9) 423–429

Lockwood G 1997 Infertility and early pregnancy loss. In: McPherson A, Waller D (eds) Women's health, 4th edn. Oxford University Press, Oxford, Ch 8

Mack S, Tucker J 1996 Counselling for the experience of infertility. In: Fertility counsellling. Baillière Tindall, London, Ch 7

Power M 1997 Fertility problems. In: Andrews G (ed) Women's sexual health. Baillière Tindall, London, Ch 8

FURTHER READING

Mack S, Tucker J 1996 Fertility counselling. Baillière Tindall, London

Furse A 1997 The infertility companion: a user's guide to tests, technology and therapies. Thorsons, London

Power M 1997 Fertility problems. In: Andrews G (ed) Women's sexual health. Baillière Tindall, London, Ch 8

RESOURCES

CHILD, The National Fertility Support Network, Charter House, 43 St Leonards Road, Bexhill on Sea, East Sussex TN40 1JA, UK. Tel.: 01424 732361.

Family Planning Association, 2–12 Pentonville Road, London N1 9FP, UK. Tel.: 020 7837 5432.

Human Fertilisation and Embryology Authority, Paxton House, 30 Artillery Lane, London E1 7LS, UK. Tel.: 020 7377 5077.

ISSUE, The National Fertility Association, 114 Lichfield Street, Walsall WS1 1SZ, UK. Tel.: 01922 722888.

ASSISTED CONCEPTION

Assisted conception is the means by which infertile or subfertile couples may be helped to achieve a pregnancy. The choice of technique will depend on the cause, or causes, of a particular couples' fertility problem. The techniques include (HFEA 1997):

- ovulation induction
- surgery to improve blocked or damaged uterine tubes
- artificial insemination using the husband's or partner's sperm
- insemination using donor sperm (DI) if the husband or partner has no sperm or very poor sperm or risks passing on an inherited disease
- in vitro fertilization (IVF)
- egg donation with IVF where the woman cannot produce eggs
- embryo donation
- gamete intra-fallopian transfer (GIFT) using the couple's own or donated sperm or eggs
- intra-cytoplasmic sperm injection (ICSI).

WHERE CAN THESE TECHNIQUES BE CARRIED OUT?

- Ovulation induction can be carried out in primary care.
- Only clinics licensed and regulated by the Human Fertilisation and Embryology Authority (HFEA) can carry out
  - IVF
  - DI
  - GIFT using donated sperm or eggs
  - storage of sperm or embryos (see p. 149).

THE TECHNIQUES
Ovulation induction

- Anti-oestrogens (clomiphene and tamoxifen)
  - increase gonadotrophin release by blocking oestrogen receptors
  - increase risk of multiple pregnancy (rarely more than twins), ultrasound monitoring is recommended
  - clomiphene should not normally be used for more than six cycles (possible increased risk of ovarian cancer)
  - both given orally
  - possible risk of ovarian hyperstimulation syndrome (OHSS).
- Gonadotrophins are indicated for women
  - with proven hypopituitarism
  - or who have not responded to clomiphene
  - in super-ovulation treatment for assisted conception (e.g. IVF)
  - given by injection
  - risk of OHSS (BNF 1998).

Donor insemination (DI)

This is carried out using sperm from a donor who has undergone HIV testing and other health screening. The sperm has been quarantined for at least 6 months (for repeat HIV tests on the donor). The procedure is carried out by placing the sperm in the woman's vagina, cervix or uterus. One or more inseminations may be carried out around the time of ovulation. Efforts are made to match the physical characteristics of the donor with the male partner. Donors are anonymous, and have no rights or responsibilities in respect of children who are born.

Gamete intra-fallopian transfer (GIFT)

Clinics using donated eggs or sperm must be licensed by the HFEA. However, the HFEA does not regulate GIFT if the woman's own eggs and the partner's sperm are used. GIFT can be used if the uterine tubes are patent or if the cause of infertility is unexplained. During the procedure eggs are retrieved, mixed with sperm and placed directly within one or other uterine tube. Up to three eggs can be transferred in any treatment cycle, to reduce the risk of a multiple birth. Fertilization takes place inside the woman's body.

In vitro fertilization (IVF)

This procedure may be appropriate if the woman has blocked uterine tubes, or the man has very few sperm. One or more eggs are retrieved from maturing follicles. Ovulation induction may have been used to produce several mature follicles. After collection, the eggs are mixed with the sperm, in a dish, and placed in an incubator to be fertilized and so produce one or more embryos. A maximum of three embryos may be placed in the woman's uterus at any one time.

Intra-cytoplasmic sperm injection (ICSI)

This is one of a number of techniques of micromanipulation and may be appropriate where the male partner has very few sperm. A single sperm is injected directly into an egg that has previously been retrieved. If the egg fertilizes, it can be transferred into the uterus in the same way as IVF.

IVF using donated eggs, sperm or embryos

These may be used if the male partner is infertile or if using donated eggs. The technique may also be used if one of the couple is at risk of passing on a serious inherited disease. It may also be used if both partners are infertile but the woman is able to carry a baby to full term. The clinic must have the appropriate facilities. Egg donors are usually women who have completed their families and are undergoing sterilization, or women who are themselves undergoing IVF treatment, or who simply wish to help others. In January 2000 the HFEA agreed to permit the use of frozen eggs in fertility treatment since the procedure is shown to be sufficiently safe. The statutory storage period is now 10 years.

Transport/satellite IVF

This procedure may be offered to those who do not live near a licensed IVF clinic. The ovulation induction and egg collection is carried out at a hospital near to the woman's home. The eggs are transported in an incubator to the licensed IVF clinic where they are fertilized. Alternatively the woman begins ovulation induction and monitoring, and then travels to the licensed IVF clinic for egg collection, fertilization and embryo transfer. The live birth rate for transport IVF is not always the same as for conventional IVF. There are guidelines for nurses working in units offering transport IVF (RCN 1996).

Embryo freezing and storage

Some clinics have storage facilities so that spare embryos can be frozen for use in a later treatment cycle if required. This facility may avoid the need for repeated drug stimulation, egg retrieval, sperm collection and fertilization. Not all embryos survive freezing and thawing and the live birth rate from frozen embryos is usually lower than for fresh embryo transfers. Any remaining embryos that are not required can be donated for the treatment of others, donated for research or allowed to perish. Genetic material cannot be stored indefinitely (HFEA 1997).

SUCCESS RATES

From 1 April 1995 to 31 March 1996:

- the average live birth rate for women of all ages (also called the 'take home baby' rate) for IVF and ICSI nation-wide was 17.4%

- the average live birth rate using embryo transfer was 21.1%
- using ICSI only the rate was 22.0%.

Some issues to consider when choosing a clinic are (HFEA 1997):

- Does the clinic have a risk of multiple birth and treatment policy? The HFEA recommends limiting the number of embryos to two to minimize the chance of triplets.
- Multiple births can lead to a much higher risk of:
  - complications during pregnancy
  - premature birth and low weight
  - disability and
  - death of infants at or within 28 days of birth (neonatal death).
- Risk of OHSS:
  - the clinic should have a policy for avoiding this
  - the patient should be aware of what signs to look out for.
- Any tests and investigations carried out on an individual should be all the tests that are necessary while avoiding duplication and understanding that unexplained infertility can be treated successfully.
- Treatments offered by clinics: the treatment must be appropriate to the individual's infertility and not all clinics offer all forms of treatment.
- Restriction on treatment: some clinics have an upper age limit for women (where the treatment is provided by the NHS, this limit is usually decided by the health authority which is paying for the treatment); some clinics do not offer treatment to single women or unmarried couples.
- Waiting lists: for consultation appointment and for treatment.
- Frequency of visits to the clinic: expense of time off work and travel.
- Patient support groups: some clinics have their own groups.
- Cost of treatment: whether or not receiving NHS treatment, if there are charges and exactly what they cover, e.g. the cost of a full treatment cycle including any additional charges for items such as drugs, consultations or embryo storage or possible refund of part of the fee if a treatment cycle is abandoned.
- NHS funding: each health authority decides what funding will be allocated to the treatment of infertility and the types of treatment offered; there are usually eligibility criteria for access to funding.

- What will happen if a pregnancy is achieved? The extent to which clinics remain involved varies.
- What will happen if a pregnancy is not achieved?:
  - advice and counselling should be offered
  - further attempts may be made
  - different type of treatment may be tried
  - may withdraw from further treatment.

Nursing issues

Spend some time thinking about the following:

- knowledge of some of the techniques used in assisted conception
- understanding the importance of support for the couple through the whole process, whatever the outcome
- knowledge of local health authority policy on assisted conception
- respecting the individual's beliefs and needs
- awareness of the intrusion into the personal and intimate life of the infertile couple
- awareness of the strain that infertility places on sexual, family and personal relationships
- awareness of social and cultural attitudes to infertility and assisted conception (Mack & Tucker 1996)
- awareness of the role of the fertility nurse specialist
- knowledge of local and national resources, support groups and information.

Some other considerations for an individual or couple considering assisted conception:

- there should be comprehensive information given using appropriate language about the treatment offered, including risks and costs
- the availability of counselling, which must be offered before proceeding with treatment
  - support counselling
  - implications counselling
  - therapeutic counselling (HFEA 1997)
- consent issues: informed consent is required, with patients and donors giving written consent to the use and storage of their sperm, the use of their eggs, and to the use and storage of any resultant embryos. Sperm, eggs and embryos can only be used with that consent, which can be changed or withdrawn at any time
- confidentiality
- who and what to tell: the experience of infertility can result in feelings of shame, guilt and blame, falling self-esteem, and a loss of femininity and masculinity (Mack & Tucker 1996). There may be pressure to produce a grandchild. Family and friends may believe that all assisted conception techniques are unnatural, especially those using donor gametes and that any child born as a result of these techniques would not 'belong' to the family

---

Nursing issues (continued)

- how to stop: some infertile couples will need to be supported in making their decision to stop trying after unsuccessful treatment, and learn how to live their lives without children
- surrogacy (see p. 68) may be a solution for some.

Key points

Ovarian hyperstimulation syndrome (OHSS):

- mild to moderate form
  - ovarian enlargement
  - abdominal distension and pain
  - can usually be treated by bedrest, fluids and simple analgesics
  - the cycle may have to be abandoned
- severe form
  - approximately 1% incidence
  - a gynaecological emergency
  - greatly enlarged ovaries with multiple follicular cysts
  - ascites and pleural effusion giving symptoms of abdominal pain, nausea and vomiting, shortness of breath
  - feeling weak and faint
  - electrolyte imbalance and reduced urine output
  - urgent hospital treatment is needed to restore fluid balance and monitor progress.

Egg donation:

- some women are offered incentives if they are able to recruit egg donors. The incentive may be earlier or cheaper treatment.

REFERENCES

BNF 1998 Hypothalamic and anterior pituitary hormones and anti-oestrogens. British National Formulary, Number 35. British Medical Association and Royal Pharmaceutical Society of Great Britain, Ch 6

HFEA 1997 The patients' guide to DI and IVF clinics, 3rd edn. Human Fertilisation and Embryology Authority, London

Mack S, Tucker J 1996 Overview of current practices in the UK and other countries. In: Fertility counselling. Baillière Tindall, London, Ch 1

RCN 1996 Transport IVF: Guideline for nurses working in units offering transport in vitro fertilisation. Royal College of Nursing, London

---

RESOURCES

CHILD (The National Infertility Support Network), Charter House, 43 St Leonards Road, Bexhill-on-Sea, East Sussex TN40 1JA, UK. Tel.: 10424 732631.

Childlessness Overcome Through Surrogacy (COTS), Loandhu Cottage, Gruids, Lairg, Sutherland IV27 4EF, UK.

ISSUE (The National Fertility Association), 114 Lichfield Street, Walsall WS1 1SZ, Tel.: 01922 722888.

NEEDS (National Egg & Embryo Donation Society), St Mary's Hospital, Whitworth Park, Manchester M13 0HJ, UK.

SEXUALLY TRANSMITTED INFECTIONS

Sexually transmitted infections (STIs) refer to any infection that can be spread through sexual activity, e.g.:

- HIV
- AIDS
- herpes
- genital warts
- syphilis
- gonorrhoea
- non-specific genital infection
- *Chlamydia*
- trichomoniasis
- candidiasis
- hepatitis B.

Some infections can be passed on without full intercourse. With some STIs there are no symptoms and following infection with some STIs there may be a long period with no symptoms. It is not uncommon for more than one STI to be present together.

The *Health of the Nation* document (DOH 1992) set targets:

- to reduce the incidence of HIV infection
- to reduce the incidence of other sexually transmitted diseases.

A reduction by at least 20% of new cases of gonorrhoea in men and women aged 15–64 by 1995 is one target that most GUM clinics appear to have achieved (Handy 1996).

SYMPTOMS

General symptoms of STIs are:

- dysuria
- vaginal discharge

- intermenstrual bleeding
- vulval soreness or irritation
- pelvic pain.

However, there may be no symptoms at all, but the woman may have reason to believe herself at risk.

MANAGEMENT

STIs should be managed by accurate diagnosis and effective treatment. A management plan should include (Adler 1995):

- sexual history
- physical examination
- microbiology
- serology
- tracing sexual contacts
- education
- reassurance
- follow-up.

Where should STIs be treated?

GPs may be able to promote safer sexual practices, take a sexual history and carry out a limited number of basic microbiological tests on their own patients and treat accordingly.

Family planning clinics may be able to promote safer sexual practices, take a sexual history and carry out a range of basic microbiological tests on anyone who chooses to access the service, but there may be limited treatment options. However, genitourinary medicine (GUM) clinics offer the best option to anyone who suspects that he or she may have or be at risk of having an STI.

GUM clinics

The advantages of GUM clinics are (Adler 1995):

- totally confidential service
- free treatment
- accessible to all by self-referral, or referral by GP or family planning clinic

- offer prompt diagnosis and treatment
- minimize the incidence of complications
- trace and treat infected partners
- educate patients, public and health care workers.

Additionally GUM clinics can offer:

- cervical screening
- HIV counselling and testing
- colposcopy
- emergency contraception
- condoms
- specialist clinics for those who are HIV positive or who have AIDS
- psychosexual problems clinics.

Some areas have Sexual Health Clinics, which are a 'one-stop-shop' providing a full range of services promoting sexual and reproductive health, including full family planning provision.

Nursing issues

Spend some time thinking about the following:

- having accurate information around STIs and sexual health
- knowledge of local and national resources and services
- taking advantage of opportunities to promote sexual health and reduce the risk of acquiring an STI
- identification of those who may be at particular risk (without making assumptions about lifestyle and class that may exclude someone from appropriate treatment)
- understanding the importance of taking an accurate sexual history
- awareness of issues of consent to testing and to treatment
- awareness of issues of confidentiality, e.g. in relation to contact tracing
- understanding of the psychological impact of an STI
- awareness of possible concerns around fertility
- awareness of one's own moral and sexual attitudes:
  'It is bad manners for staff to force their own attitudes on a patient and it is also bad medicine, since the patient will not come back.' (Adler 1995)
- awareness of issues around sexuality
- ensuring access to the most appropriate treatment
- specialist nurses can provide sensitive and supportive holistic care, while carrying out a wide range of diagnostic and treatment procedures.

OTHER CONSIDERATIONS

When taking a sexual history the nurse should (Nash 1997):

- ensure the woman understands why it is necessary
- recognize the personal and sensitive nature of issues involved
- recognize own feelings (embarrassment, attitudes, beliefs and values) that can influence the nature of the consultation
- use appropriate language for that woman, possibly street language
- listen carefully, observing non-verbal communication
- ask purposeful questions
- do not make assumptions or judgements about lifestyle or sexuality (refer to partner as 'partner' and not by gender, e.g. 'husband')
- work within professional boundaries and framework of the law (e.g. in relation to consent and confidentiality)
- always protect the woman's right to confidentiality.

Some issues it may be appropriate to follow up after treatment for an STI are:

- Was the diagnosis confirmed?
- Has the correct treatment been given?
- Has the treatment been taken?
- Is a follow-up necessary?
- What about sexual contacts?
- What about future fertility?
- What about the impact of an STI on personal and sexual relationships?
- How can that woman protect herself?
- Are there issues of coercion or abuse?

Reducing the risk of contracting a sexually transmitted infection is achieved by the following (Adler 1997):

- abstain
- avoid multiple partners, prostitutes and other people with multiple sex partners
- avoid sexual contact with people who have symptoms or lesions (e.g. urethral discharge, warts, ulcers)
- avoid genital contact with oral 'cold sores'
- use condoms or diaphragm
- have regular check-ups if at higher risk of STIs.

Think about the sexual health needs of some women:

- The woman who believes she is in a monogamous relationship.
- The young woman who has a learning disability.
- The disabled woman in a wheelchair.
- The woman who is bisexual.
- The woman whose partner is bisexual.
- The woman who knows that her partner is promiscuous, but believes him when he says that she won't catch anything from him.

There now follows a brief outline of the most commonly encountered STIs, including the incidence, symptoms, diagnosis, management and treatment. Full references, further reading and resources follow at the end of the chapter.

> **Key points**
>
> - Anyone can get STIs, whatever their class, education, etc.
> - There is still stigma attached to acquiring STIs.
> - Caring for those with, or at risk of, an STI is so sensitive and important that the care best comes only from those who are appropriately trained.

BACTERIAL VAGINOSIS

Bacterial vaginosis (BV) is the commonest cause of vaginal symptoms in women of childbearing age. It is an overgrowth of naturally occurring vaginal bacteria, where the normal lactobacilli of the vagina are replaced, usually with *Gardnerella vaginalis* and mixed anaerobes. There is no agreement on whether the condition is sexually transmitted; although it is more common in women who are currently sexually active, it can occur in women who are not currently sexually active. It may be significantly more common among lesbians (Phillips et al 1996).

Symptoms

Up to half of women with BV will have no symptoms. Those that do experience the following:

- an increase in vaginal discharge, typically grey/white and watery

- a strong fishy-smelling discharge, particularly after sexual intercourse
- occasionally there may be itching in or around the vagina.

Causes

Possibly by any agent that raises the pH of the vagina, including:

- menstrual blood
- semen
- vaginal douching
- vaginal deodorants
- strongly scented soaps, bubble bath, etc.
- strong detergents (especially 'biological') to wash underwear
- intrauterine device (IUD), in some women, is associated with recurrent BV (Sonnex 1997).

However, BV frequently develops without any of these conditions.

Diagnosis

- Classic thin grey/white vaginal discharge.
- pH of discharge >4.5.
- Positive 'whiff' test – when potassium hydroxide is added to a sample of discharge there is a characteristic fishy smell.
- Presence of clue cells on microscopy (vaginal epithelial cells with adherent anaerobic bacteria).

Three of the four indicators must be found for a diagnosis of BV to be made. In GUM clinics the result of the tests may be available immediately. There may be no indication to treat a healthy, asymptomatic woman (Phillips et al 1996). BV may be a marker for other STIs (Bradbeer 1997)

Treatment

- Metronidazole tablets.
- Clindamycin vaginal cream.
- Treatment of sexual partners does not improve the recurrence rate for women, but they should probably be treated if the woman has recurrent attacks (Phillips et al 1996).

BV and pregnancy

BV in pregnancy is associated with:

- premature rupture of the membranes
- premature labour and birth
- post-partum endometritis.

Metronidazole is contraindicated in the first trimester of pregnancy, in which case the condition is treated with clindamycin.

CANDIDIASIS (THRUSH)

Candidiasis is the commonest organism causing a vaginal discharge. It is an infection caused by a yeast-like fungus, usually *Candida albicans*. *Candida* can normally be found in the mouth, gut and vagina. It thrives in warm, moist conditions and is present in the vaginas of 20% of women with no symptoms. *Candida* only appears to become pathogenic under certain conditions. It is not generally sexually transmitted, but is associated with other sexually acquired conditions in >30% of cases (Adler 1995). As many as 75% of women will have at least one episode of vaginal thrush at some time in their lives (Phillips et al 1996).

Triggers

Common triggers are (Adler 1995):

- pregnancy
- antibiotic treatment
- corticosteroid treatment
- immunosuppressive treatment
- diabetes
- the presence of other STIs
- immune deficiencies (e.g. HIV disease).

Other associated factors are:

- poor personal hygiene
  - keep the genital area clean and dry
  - avoid nylon pants, tights and jeans

- always wipe genitalia from front to back (to avoid spreading bacteria from the bowel)
- trauma to the vaginal mucosa
  - during sexual intercourse
  - by douching, or using vaginal deodorants, perfumed soaps, bubble bath, etc.
  - by using vaginal tampons during menstruation.

Symptoms

- Itching and soreness of the vagina and vulva.
- Inflammation and oedema of the vagina and vulva.
- A thick, white discharge (looking like cottage cheese).
- Dysuria.
- Dyspareunia (pain with sex).

Diagnosis

Clinical examination is notoriously unreliable for diagnosis, but culture and microscopy of a high vaginal or cervical swab may reveal its presence. *Candida* may occasionally be diagnosed on a routine cervical smear (Oakeshott 1997).

Treatment

Treatment is only recommended if the woman is symptomatic:

- antifungal vaginal pessaries +/– cream (clotrimazole or miconazole)
- oral antifungal tablet (fluconazole – contraindicated in pregnancy or lactation).

Recurrent candidiasis:

- can be difficult to manage
- other infection must be excluded
- male partners should be investigated
- known triggers should be avoided
- prophylaxis may be advised
- can cause sexual and relationship difficulties.

> **Key points**
>
> - High oestrogen oral contraceptive pills were thought to cause candidiasis.
> - The lower dose pills currently in use are not believed to cause candidiasis (Phillips et al 1996).

CHLAMYDIA

Chlamydia is an infection caused by the bacteria *Chlamydia trachomatis*. It is probably the most common STI: prevalence is 2–12% in general practice populations. Untreated infection significantly affects male and female fertility.

The infection is usually in the endocervix, but can also spread to the endometrium, uterine tubes, peritoneum, rectum and urethra, causing inflammation, ulceration and scarring (Nash 1997).

Treatment is simple and effective, once a diagnosis has been made; accurate diagnosis is best carried out in a GUM clinic.

Symptoms

Up to 70% of women have no symptoms (Oakeshott 1997). Others may experience mild symptoms of

- vaginal discharge
- intermenstrual bleeding
- lower abdominal pain
- dysuria.

Chlamydia may cause pelvic inflammatory disease (PID) (see p. 314).

Diagnosis

The most commonly used technique is taking a specimen from the cervix containing endocervical cells, since *Chlamydia* is an intracellular bacterium. The sample should not contain pus or discharge, which should have been cleaned off the cervix.

No one test is totally reliable and each test is as good as the skill of the clinician. Any pelvic examination that is carried out at the same time may be normal. However, mucopurulent vaginal discharge may be present, and the cervix may be friable, bleeding easily on contact.

Treatment

- Doxycycline 100 mg orally twice daily for 7 days.
- Erythromycin 500 mg four times a day for 7 days, if pregnant or lactating.
- Contact tracing and treatment of partner is essential.
- Abstaining from sex until partner has been treated (or using a condom if this is not possible).

Follow-up tests are usually only required if there are doubts about partner's compliance with treatment. The promotion of good sexual health practices is essential.

GUIDELINES

Although treatment of uncomplicated infection is cheap and cost-effective, *Chlamydia* infection is often poorly managed. The Central Audit Group in Genitourinary Medicine (1998) has produced guidelines for the management of *Chlamydia* (*Clinical Guidelines and Standards for the Management of Uncomplicated Genital Chlamydia Infection*), with standards for:

- diagnosis
- treatment
- follow-up
- management of contacts
- standards for partner notification.

These guidelines are for use in GUM clinics, but may be useful in other settings. The general principles are transferable for other infections.

Chlamydia and the neonate

Between 30 and 50% of infants born to women with *Chlamydia* will develop eye disease that can resolve spontaneously (this may be the first sign that the woman is infected). While 10–20% of babies will develop pneumonia through the inhalation of infected material during birth, symptoms usually present 1–3 months after birth (Adler 1995).

Chlamydia and fertility

The first sign that a woman has had *Chlamydia* may be when she presents with infertility. *Chlamydia* can persist in the cervix for years and is the major organism found in PID. PID and tubal damage is a significant cause of infertility.

Screening

Screening programmes, notably in Sweden, have significantly reduced the prevalence of chlamydia and PID. In 1998 two sites were chosen, in the UK, to pilot a chlamydia screening programme. The pilot sites are targetting those considered at high risk, by age or other factors. To be an effective screening programme testing should be available to *all* sexually active women of reproductive age. Screening tests are expensive, but the cost of investigating and treating infertility is far more costly.

Key points

- Infection with chlamydia is more common:
  - in sexually active women under 25 years of age
  - when not using either contraception or barrier method of contraception
  - if the women has had two or more sexual partners in last year
  - with a partner who has had gonorrhoea or non-specific urethritis (NSU) (Nash 1997).
- Indications for *Chlamydia* testing (Oakeshott 1997):
  - mucopurulent vaginal discharge
  - suspected PID
  - suspected STI
  - before termination of pregnancy (TOP)
  - before insertion of intrauterine contraceptive device (IUCD)
  - sexually active teenagers.

GENITAL WARTS

Genital warts are caused by the human papillomavirus (HPV). They are nearly always transmitted by sexual contact. Autoinoculation from hand to genitals is unusual, but can occur. Infectivity from a symptomatically infected sexual partner is 60%. The incubation period varies from 2 weeks to 8 months, with an average of 3 months, and is frequently associated with one or more additional infections (Adler 1995).

Once HPV is in the person's body, it is there for life. A first attack is most commonly in the 20–24 year age group (Phillips et al 1996). A sudden first attack does not automatically suggest infidelity (Husband 1996).

Symptoms

Genital warts are frequently asymptomatic and painless, although they may cause itching. They flourish in warm, moist conditions, particularly if a discharge or other infections are present. The commonest site in women is the introitus and vulva, also the perineum. They can also be found in the vagina and on the cervix. Anal warts can develop without having had anal sex.

How long do they last?

Genital warts may spontaneously regress, but they can also increase considerably in pregnancy, old age and in people who are immunosuppressed (Nash 1997). Once infected, people may transmit the virus to others – even when they themselves are asymptomatic. It is not known if they remain infectious for ever (Oakeshott 1997).

Diagnosis

Diagnosis is by:

- clinical examination
- subclinical infection, which is frequently diagnosed on routine cervical smear.

Treatment

Since it is impossible to eradicate the virus, current treatment is to remove the warts, usually by using podophyllin:

- a cytotoxic resin that is painted onto the warts
  - it is applied once or twice a week for up to 4 weeks
  - it can cause burning and local irritation
  - it cannot be used in pregnancy.

Alternative treatments include:

- stronger local agents

- cryotherapy
- electrocautery
- surgical excision.

Key points

- There are many different types of HPV.
- Certain types have a strong association with cervical intraepithelial neoplasia (CIN) (see p. 339).
- Flat warts on the cervix are not usually visible to the naked eye.
- Women with vulval warts, or whose partners have warts, should have a colposcopy (see p. 328) to exclude cervical warts.
- Regular cervical screening is recommended.
- Other STIs must be excluded.
- Contact tracing must be carried out.
- Safer sexual practices, including condom use, must be discussed.

GONORRHOEA

Gonorrhoea, one of the venereal diseases, is a bacterial infection of the mucous membranes. It is caused by the organism *Neisseria gonorrhoeae* and is highly contagious, being passed on by intimate contact, sexual intercourse and oral sex.

It most commonly affects the cervix, urethra, rectum and oropharynx.

Colloquially known as 'the clap', gonorrhoea has an incubation period of 3 to 7 days. Many of those infected will have no symptoms. It is often associated with other STIs, particularly trichomonas and chlamydia. Rectal infection can occur without anal intercourse, by infection from vaginal secretions (Nash 1997).

After some years of decline it is now on the increase in some areas of England and Wales in teenage women and young adult men, particularly those from black minority groups (Low et al 1997). It can cause salpingitis and pelvic inflammatory disease (PID) (p. 314). Damage to the uterine tubes can cause ectopic pregnancy and infertility, while infection in pregnancy can result in the baby having gonococcal conjunctivitis. More strains are now penicillin-resistant, particularly when contracted in other countries.

Signs and symptoms

- There may be no symptoms in 40% of those affected.
- Men are more likely to have symptoms than women.
- Most common symptoms are (Hardy 1996):
  - purulent vaginal discharge
  - dysuria and frequency
  - urethral discharge
  - cervicitis
  - intermenstrual bleeding.

Diagnosis

Swabs are taken for microscopy and culture, usually from the cervix and urethra, and possibly the rectum. An endocervical swab will diagnose gonorrhoea in 90% of cases (Adler 1995).

Treatment and management

This is carried out by means of accurate diagnosis and exclusion of other STIs.

Antibiotic treatment can be a single dose, but that will depend on:

- local drug resistance pattern
- pregnancy
- drug sensitivity/allergy
- other infection.

Contact tracing is essential, as is abstinence from sexual intercourse. Swabs should be repeated following treatment to confirm the effectiveness of that treatment (the 'test of cure') (Handy 1996).

HEPATITIS B

Hepatitis B is one of five recognized hepatitis viruses. A sexually transmitted infection, it is the only hepatitis likely to be spread by both heterosexual and homosexual sex. It can also be spread through other body fluids, e.g. blood, saliva and urine. Those at high risk of infection include homosexual men and injecting drug misusers. The infection has an incubation period from 1 to 6 months.

Hepatitis B can cause long-term liver damage and the possible development of cirrhosis, which is associated with a high risk of primary hepatocellular carcinoma (Adler 1995).

Treatment

There is a lack of effective treatment, therefore, prevention is vital in controlling the disease by:

- promoting safer sexual practices (see p. 48)
- active immunization
- contact tracing.

Key points

Think about the woman:

- who is a drug misuser
- whose partner is bisexual and/or a drug misuser
- who comes from a country where hepatitis B is endemic.

GENITAL HERPES

Genital herpes, the commonest cause of genital ulcers, is caused by the herpes simplex virus (HSV). HSV is categorized into types 1 and 2. Both types cause genital infection, but type 1 usually causes cold sores on the face and lips.

HSV can be transmitted by oro-genital contact, and is frequently transmitted by those who do not know they are infected or who are asymptomatic (Oakeshott 1997).

Why is it a problem?

It is a problem because (Adler 1995):

- the incidence is increasing
- it is the fourth commonest STI
- it is incurable
- it is recurrent
- it can lead to a breakdown of relationships, psychosexual problems and depression
- it may cause neonatal and possibly fetal infections.

Symptoms

First attack (Adler 1995)

- There is a short incubation period of less than 7 days.
- Usual presentation is multiple, very painful genital ulcers.
- Occasionally there may be no symptoms.
- There is usually painful, enlarged inguinal lymph nodes.
- The ulcers gradually scab over and heal, leaving no scarring.
- Systemic symptoms include fever and malaise.
- The cervix and vulva are usually affected (in 80–90% of cases).
- Buttocks, thighs and anus may also be affected.
- Micturition can be extremely painful.
- The virus is shed from the lesions until healing is complete, usually about 12 days.
- The whole illness may last 3 weeks.

Recurrent attacks

Less than 50% of those affected will have recurrent attacks. These are less severe and not due to reinfection. Infection with type 2 HSV produces recurrences earlier after the primary infection than type 1 HSV. More than 50% of those infected have no symptoms for the first or recurrent attacks.

In recurrent attacks the symptoms are milder and of shorter duration, lasting 8–10 days, and there are usually no systemic symptoms. There is often itching, tingling or numbness at the site 24 to 48 hours before a recurrence (these are called prodromal symptoms). Reported precipitating causes for recurrences include (Adler 1995):

- stress
- sexual intercourse
- menstruation/hormonal changes
- climatic changes (heat/cold)

Diagnosis

Diagnosis:

- is by clinical examination
- is by viral culture, from a vesicle or from an ulcer
- other STIs must be excluded

- if the woman has travelled abroad recently or if her partner is from abroad then tropical ulcers must be excluded
- there are some non-sexually transmitted causes of genital ulceration.

Treatment and management

Good management, that includes accurate diagnosis and counselling, can reduce the physical and psychological effects associated with the condition (McDermott 1996).

Primary attack

Main treatment aim:

- promoting comfort
- promoting healing
- preventing secondary infection
- decreasing transmission of the disease.

Using:

- warm saline to bathe the lesions
- mild analgesia (paracetamol)
- oral aciclovir (previously acyclovir), an antiviral:
  - treatment to start after the onset of symptoms
  - prevents viral replication
  - may reduce the duration and severity of symptoms
  - is not a cure
  - has no effect on recurrence rates
- abstinence from sexual intercourse until all the ulcers have healed, since a condom will not always prevent contact with an infected area (Nash 1997)
- contact tracing
- counselling.

Recurrent attacks

Treatment of recurrent attacks is by:

- reassurance and advice about avoiding trigger factors
- recognition of prodromal symptoms
- guidance about managing symptoms

- awareness of the need for condom use, since viral shedding can exist between overt attacks (Adler 1995)
- awareness of need for abstinence during an attack
- antiviral treatment
  - cream may help mild recurrence
  - oral treatment is most effective for recurrent episodes
  - continuous therapy can be recommended for frequent attacks (more than eight a year)
- on-going support and counselling
- the frequency of recurrences usually decreases (McDermott 1996).

HSV and cervical cancer

Despite there being no compelling evidence that HSV causes cervical intraepithelial neoplasia (CIN) (see p. 339) and cancer, indefinite annual cervical smears can be unnecessarily recommended, further adding to the woman's anxiety (Foster 1995, McDermott 1996, Nash 1997).

Key points

- Hospital admission may be necessary for
  - uncontrollable pain
  - acute urinary retention
  - suspected meningitis.
- Caesarian section is advised if there are active lesions in the vagina or vulva at the end of pregnancy.

HUMAN IMMUNODEFICIENCY VIRUS (HIV)

HIV is a retrovirus that, in particular attacks, T-helper cells (also called CD4 cells), so reducing the immune response. It is infectious, being spread through the following routes:

- sexually
- vertically (during pregnancy and delivery, in breast milk)
- by intravenous drug use
- iatrogenically (e.g. by blood transfusion, organ transplant, sperm donation).

The presence of other sexually transmitted infections (STIs) appears to allow easier transmission of the virus.

HIV is incurable, but some treatments can slow down the progression of HIV infection. In the UK it is most commonly seen in gay/bisexual men and intravenous drug users. However, the incidence in heterosexual women is rising, and worldwide it is most commonly transmitted by heterosexual sex.

Acquired immune deficiency syndrome (AIDS) may develop in people who have been infected with HIV. Treatment is available for opportunistic infection only. There is frequently prejudice and stigma attached to a diagnosis of HIV infection (Hale & Sutton 1996), e.g.:

- some have brought it on themselves through their sexuality, or by taking part in high-risk activities (prostitution, drug misuse)
- some are seen as blameless victims (via contaminated blood products, infected babies)
- some are in a 'wrong' relationship (being unaware that their partner is bisexual).

Management issues

- HIV testing including pre- and post-test counselling (see below).
- HIV testing in pregnancy.
- Contact tracing and partner notification.
- Education around safer sexual practices.
- Issues of confidentiality.
- Issues around fertility (the infected woman who wants a baby; donor sperm is now frozen and stored for 3 months until it is established that the donor is not infected).
- On-going counselling and support from specialists.
- Awareness of issues around employment, housing, insurance and travel.

Guidelines for HIV testing

The HIV Nursing Society (RCN 1994) has produced a framework for pre- and post-test counselling, including:

- general principles for good practice
- aims of pre-test counselling

- to provide clients with the knowledge they need to give informed consent to the test, which may have considerable consequences for the individual concerned
- to give clients the opportunity to discuss confidentially the ways in which they can adjust their behaviour to minimize the risk of becoming infected with HIV and to avoid infecting others
- to prepare for the responsibility of a positive result
- aims of post-test counselling:
  - help understand the test result
  - assist with shock or emotional response to the result
  - provide information and personal support
  - help decide who and how to tell
  - arrange follow-up appointments
  - ensure that clients are 'never told on a Friday'.

Key point

Safer sex can be practised by:

- using appropriate condoms and lubrication for vaginal and anal intercourse
- avoiding oral sex when there are ulcers or bleeding gums
- eliminating other STIs
- using contraception appropriate to that individual.

TRICHOMONIASIS

Trichomoniasis is an infection caused by a flagellated protozoan called *Trichomonas vaginalis* (TV). It is almost always sexually transmitted. The incubation period is between 3 and 21 days.

Symptoms

Symptoms are:

- vaginal discharge
  - green-yellow, thin and frothy
  - may have a musty/fishy smell
  - usually worse after a period
  - may be profuse
- vulval inflammation, soreness and itchiness

- dysuria and frequency
- dyspareunia.

Diagnosis

Diagnosis:

- is by clinical history
- is on samples taken from the posterior fornix
  - there are microscopic techniques that can give an immediate result
  - incubation in culture medium takes a minimum of 48 hours
- of TV may be coincidental on a cervical cytology smear
- rarely, on examination the cervix may have a 'strawberry' appearance caused by small punctate haemorrhages.

Treatment

Usual treatment for TV infection:

- metronidazole, an antimicrobial drug that is highly effective against anaerobic bacteria and protozoa, warning that metronidazole can cause nausea
- metronidazole may be teratogenic and should not be used in first trimester of pregnancy
- tracing and treating sexual contacts is essential
- abstain from sex until treatment and follow-up check completed.

Key points

- Women with TV are frequently asymptomatic.
- Other STIs are frequently found as well: 19% also have gonorrhoea (Adler 1995).
- Can be common in pregnancy, also affecting the urinary tract.
- The infection can be passed on non-sexually through moist towels and flannels; this is rare.

REFERENCES

Adler MW (ed) 1995 ABC of sexually transmitted diseases. BMJ Publishing, London

Bradbeer C 1997 Sexually transmitted disease. In: Luesley D (ed) Common conditions in gynaecology. Chapman & Hall, London, Ch 6

Central Audit Group in Genitourinary Medicine 1998 Clinical guidelines and standards for the management of uncomplicated genital chlamydia infection. Health Education Authority, London

Department of Health 1992 Health of the nation. HMSO, London

Foster P 1995 Cancer screening. In: Women and the health care industry: an unhealthy partnership? Open University Press, Buckingham, Ch 6

Hale J, Sutton A 1996 HIV and AIDS. In: Sutton A, Payne S (eds) Genito-urinary medicine for nurses. Whurr, London, Ch 10

Handy P 1996 Gonorrhoea and non-specific urethritis. In: Sutton A, Payne S (eds) Genito-urinary medicine for nurses. Whurr, London, Ch 5

Husband P 1996 Genital warts. In: Sutton A, Payne S (eds) Genito-urinary medicine for nurses. Whurr, London, Ch 8

Low N, Daker-White G, Barlow D, Pozniak A 1997 Gonorrhoea in inner London: results of a cross sectional study. British Medical Journal 314: 1719–1723

McDermott G 1996 Genital herpes and molluscum contagiosum. In: Sutton A, Payne S (eds) Genito-urinary medicine for nurses. Whurr, London, Ch 9

Nash J 1997 Sexual health and sexually acquired infection. In: Andrews G (ed) Women's sexual health. Baillière Tindall, London, Ch 12

Oakeshott P 1997 Vaginal discharge and sexually transmitted diseases. In: McPherson A, Waller D (eds) Women's health, 4th edn. Oxford University Press, Oxford, Ch 13

Phillips M, McGlynn C and Fagan B 1996 Bacterial vaginosis, candidiasis and trichomoniasis. In: Sutton A, Payne S (eds) Genito-urinary medicine for nurses. Whurr, London, Ch 7

RCN 1994 AIDS/HIV infection nursing guidelines, 2nd edn. HIV Nursing Society, Royal College of Nursing, London

Sonnex C 1997 Contraception and urogenital infection. Trends in Urology, Gynaecology and Sexual Health, September 29–32, 37

FURTHER READING

Adler M (ed) 1995 ABC of sexually transmitted diseases, 3rd edn. BMJ Publishing, London

Carter Y, Moss A, Weyman A (eds) 1998 RCGP handbook of sexual health in primary care. Royal College of General Practitioners, London

Nash J 1997 Sexual health and sexually acquired infection. In: Andrews G (ed) Women's sexual health. Baillière Tindall, London

Sutton A, Payne S (eds) 1996 Genito-urinary medicine for nurses. Whurr, London

RESOURCES

Health Education Authority, 30 Great Peter Street, London SW1, UK. Tel.: 020 7222 5300.

Herpes Virus Association (Sphere), 41 North Road, London N7 9PD, UK. Tel.: 020 7609 9061 (helpline).

National AIDS Helpline, Tel.: 0800 567 123.

Positively Women, 347 City Road, London EC1, UK. Tel.: 020 7713 0222 (helpline).

This chapter explores some of the issues that are particularly relevant to the mature woman. The menopause, by definition the end of menstruation, is exclusive to women. Osteoporosis is experienced by a small number of men, but is much more of a female condition, resulting in considerable morbidity and mortality. Cardiovascular disease is generally seen as a male problem; consequently it is frequently under-diagnosed and under-treated in postmenopausal women.

HORMONE REPLACEMENT THERAPY

Hormone replacement therapy (HRT) is the use of oestrogen to replace that lost as the result of ovarian failure. A woman who has had a hysterectomy may be given oestrogen alone. Those women who have an intact uterus (i.e. have not had a hysterectomy) must have the oestrogen 'opposed' with progestogen to prevent endometrial hyperplasia, which can be a precursor for endometrial cancer (Redman 1997).

An alternative for some women is a gonadomimetic, a synthetic preparation with oestrogenic, progestogenic and androgenic properties.

More recently, selective oestrogen receptor modulators (SERMs), which have 'anti-oestrogen' effects, have been developed. One of them, raloxifene, has been approved for osteoporosis prevention.

The menopause is a natural event; however, the medical model can emphasize the 'deficiency' of this natural process. Equally, because it is a natural event, many women are told that they have to accept whatever happens to them as part of women's lot.

Nursing issues

Spend some time thinking about the following:

- knowledge of the short- and long-term consequences of oestrogen deficiency
- awareness of the preparations available
- understanding of the relative and absolute contraindications to HRT
- awareness of the risks and benefits of HRT
- enabling access to therapy for those who want it
- promoting a healthy lifestyle
- promoting the advantages of HRT to those who may most benefit
- awareness of alternatives to HRT and any supporting research
- awareness that HRT can be considered as 'unnatural'
- understanding that cross-culturally the menopause can be seen as a very positive event
- understanding that there are negative attitudes to women and ageing, which need to be examined
- how specialist nurses can support women to take control for themselves
- how specialist nurses can improve compliance with taking HRT (Brown 1997).

BENEFITS OF HRT

The benefits of HRT are:

- Significant relief of some menopausal symptoms, especially hot flushes, sweats, irritability, insomnia and vaginal dryness (Whitehead & Godfree 1992).
- Prevention of osteoporosis and reduction in risk of fracture of hip, wrist and spine (NOS/RCN 1996).
- Reduction of the risk of cardiovascular disease (see p. 200) (Stampfer & Colditz 1991).
- Possible reduction of the risk of some dementias, e.g. Alzheimer's disease (Paganini-Hill 1996).
- Effective relief of short- and medium-term symptoms of the menopause (see p. 185).
- Reduction in rate of bone loss.
- A Possible increase in bone density, even in established osteoporosis.
- Associated with a 50% reduction in the incidence of osteoporotic hip fracture and associated mortality.
- Associated with a 60% reduction in mortality from ischaemic heart disease and stroke.
- Associated with a small fall in blood pressure.
- Lower incidence of endometrial cancer (Payne 1997).

RISKS OF HRT

A comprehensive evaluation of data from 51 studies on breast cancer and HRT (Collaborative Group on Hormonal Factors in Breast Cancer 1997) reached the following conclusions:

- Of women aged 50 not using HRT, 45 in every 1000 will have cancer diagnosed over the next 20 years.
- Women who use HRT for a short time around the menopause have a very low additional risk.
- Use of HRT for 5 years produces 2 extra cancers per 1000 women.
- Use of HRT for 10 years produces 6 extra cancers per 1000.
- Use of HRT for 15 years produces 12 extra cancers per 1000.
- The increased risk of breast cancer disappears within about 5 years of stopping HRT.

- Breast cancers are found earlier in women on HRT, and are easier to treat.

WHO SHOULD TAKE HRT?

- Any woman who suffers from the short-term effects of oestrogen deficiency, having vasomotor, musculoskeletal, genitourinary or psychological symptoms.
- Those women who are at particular risk of the long-term consequences of oestrogen deficiency:
  - premature menopause
  - hysterectomy before the menopause
  - had a fracture
  - history of ischaemic heart disease
  - at increased risk of osteoporosis
  - prolonged use of high dose corticosteroids (>7.5 mg daily).

CONTRAINDICATIONS TO HRT

The absolute contraindications are:

- endometrial cancer
- breast cancer
- known or suspected pregnancy
- undiagnosed abnormal vaginal bleeding
- severe, active liver disease with abnormal liver function tests
- active thromboembolic disorder (Whitehead & Godfree 1992).

There are relative contraindications to HRT and women who have certain conditions should be monitored closely after starting treatment:

- endometriosis or fibroids
- gall bladder disease
- migraine
- history of breast nodules or fibrocystic disease
- untreated hypertension.

Product literature advises caution in other conditions, including:

- obesity
- cardiac or renal disease
- hypertension
- asthma

- epilepsy
- diabetes
- hyperlipidaemia
- otosclerosis
- melanoma
- multiple sclerosis
- systemic lupus erythematosus.

Evidence for caution in these conditions is unsatisfactory, however, and many women with these conditions may stand to benefit from HRT (BNF 1998).

There is a risk of expectations of long-term protection not being met (Hannaford 1998):

- Taking HRT for too short a time.
- Not taking HRT at age of greatest risk of cardiovascular events, in the 60s.
- Most studies on the cardioprotective effects of HRT were conducted on oestrogen alone.

THINKING ABOUT HRT?

Fully counselling a woman before she starts taking HRT greatly improves continuation rate and level of satisfaction. There is a large drop-out rate for continuance after the initial consultation. Women need to be aware that not all forms of HRT suit everyone, that there are a number of choices and that it is worth persevering for some months before stopping or trying a different formulation. The following issues should be covered in the initial consultation:

- Information about the menopause and oestrogen deficiency.
- Information about the advantages and disadvantages of HRT.
- Current information about the risks and benefits.
- Exploration of individual needs and expectations.
- Possible side-effects.
- Choice of route.
- Possibility of tailoring a regimen to suit that individual.
- Length of therapy (see p. 180).
- Resumption of periods.
- Information about significance of bleeding pattern.
- Lifestyle issues.

TREATMENT

Duration of treatment

How long to take HRT for depends on the type and severity of the symptoms the woman is experiencing (BNF 1998):

- For vaginal atrophy (using a vaginal cream or pessary) – a few weeks.
- For vasomotor symptoms – at least one year.
- Early menopause – until the age of at least 50 and possibly for a further 10 years.
- Long-term for a woman without a uterus – at least 10 years.
- Long-term for a woman with a uterus – less clear since the progestogen may blunt the protective effect of low-dose oestrogen against myocardial infarction and stroke.

Preparations

Preparations can be:

- oral
- transdermal (patches or gel)
- subcutaneous implant
- vaginal (cream, pessary or tablet).

Oestrogen

Oestrogen therapy can be as:

- implant
- oral, alone or with progestogen continuously or sequentially
- gel
- patch, alone or with progestogen
- vaginal cream, pessary or tablet.

Oestrogen in HRT is 'natural', quite different from synthetic oestrogen used in oral contraception. Some continuous–combined preparations provide 'bleed-free' HRT.

Progestogen

Progestogen treatment can be:

- oral, alone or combined with oestrogen

- patch, combined with oestrogen
- progestogen releasing intrauterine system (IUS) (p. 118) will probably become licensed for use in HRT.

Gonadomimetics

Facts about gonadomimetics:

- tibolone is available in tablet form
- combines oestrogenic and progestogenic activity with weak androgenic activity
- taken continuously, without cyclical progestogen
- not to be used premenopausally
- not to be used until 12 months after the menopause
- 'period-free' HRT.

Side effects (Box 6.1)

Progestogen must be used for at least 10–12 days per month to protect the endometrium in a woman who has not had a hysterectomy. Any other regimen should be carried out at a specialist centre.

Selective oestrogen receptor modulators (SERMs)

These are described as 'anti-oestrogen'. One of these, raloxifene, is licensed for the prevention of osteoporosis and has a significant effect on bone density. Raloxifene does not appear to increase a woman's existing risk of breast cancer, nor does it significantly affect endometrial thickness. It reduces total and low-density lipoprotein (LDL) cholesterol. Unfortunately, it does not relieve vasomotor symptoms (Delmas et al 1997).

Box 6.1 Side effects of HRT

Oestrogenic	*Progestogenic*
• breast tenderness	• PMS-type symptoms
• leg cramps	• irritability
• nausea	• acne
• fluid retention	• fluid retention
• vaginal discharge	• headaches
	• breast tenderness

Routes of administration

There are advantages and disadvantages for each route, with the choice of route being up to the individual woman, as far as possible. Non-oral routes avoid the 'first pass' effect of the liver, which can affect the metabolism of oestrogens (first-pass effect is the process by which many drugs are partially inactivated on passage through the liver; some drugs may become inactive). The choice depends on whether or not the woman has had a hysterectomy, whether there is a need for systemic or local therapy. Other considerations are the woman's ability to tolerate withdrawal bleeds, and any history of skin reaction to patches (Payne 1997).

WHEN TO START HRT

Starting HRT will depend on when the woman wants to, and on an individual woman's reasons. Some women start HRT during the perimenopause, before their periods have stopped. Some women only start when they are very bothered with menopausal symptoms. Some women delay starting until they are in their 60s or later. It is never too late to start.

What investigations are needed before starting HRT?

Investigations should be:

- weight/height measurement
- blood pressure measurement
- cervical smear (if due)
- breast awareness (see p. 30)
- mammogram (if due)
- serum cholesterol (if appropriate)
- lifestyle advice
- pelvic examination (possibly) (p. 51).

SIGNIFICANCE OF BLEEDING PATTERN

Irregular bleeding is not uncommon during first few months on all regimens. Reasons for this include poor compliance, poor absorption (due to enzyme-inducing drugs, antibiotics, diarrhoea and vomiting, etc.) and possibly poor adhesion of a patch. Irregular bleeding may be due to too little/too much progestogen or too little/too much oestrogen. Bleeding may possibly also be due to pelvic pathology (fibroid, endometriosis, cervical or endometrial polyp, endometrial hyperplasia, endometrial cancer, cervical cancer).

Key points

- Some specialist centres will use HRT for women who have had treatment for breast cancer, believing, in certain circumstances, that the benefits outweigh the risks.
- Bleeding pattern must be monitored regularly.
- When the bleeding occurs is significant, since timing of bleeding can indicate if the likely cause is pharmacology or pathology.
- Persisting abnormal bleeding must be investigated.

REFERENCES

BNF 1998 Endocrine System. British National Formulary, p 317–318
Brown V 1997 The menopause and HRT: a more positive view? Nursing Standard 12 (10) 37–39
Collaborative Group on Hormonal Factors in Breast Cancer 1997 Breast cancer and hormone replacement therapy: a re-analysis of data from 51 epidemiological studies of 52 705 women with breast cancer and 108 411 women without breast cancer. Lancet 349: 120–123
Delmas M, Bjarnson N, Mitlak B et al 1997 Effects of raloxifene on bone mineral density, serum cholesterol concentrations and uterine endometrium in post menopausal women. New England Journal of Medicine 337: 1641–1647
Hannaford P 1998 Is there sufficient evidence for us to encourage the widespread use of hormone replacement therapy to prevent disease? British Journal of General Practice, February: 951–952
NOS/RCN 1996 Osteoporosis Resource Pack: for nurses, midwives and health visitors. National Osteoporosis Society.
Paganini-Hill A 1996 Oestrogen replacement therapy and Alzheimer's disease. British Journal of Obstetrics and Gynaecology 103, supplement 13, 80–86
Payne E 1997 Menopausal problems. In: Luesley D (ed) Common conditions in gynaecology. Chapman & Hall, London, Ch 13
Redman C 1997 Gynaecological cancers. In: Luesley D (ed) Common conditions in gynaecology. Chapman & Hall, London, Ch 10
Stampfer M, Colditz B 1991 Oestrogen replacement therapy and coronary heart disease: a quantitative assessment of the epidemiological evidence. Preventive Medicine 20: 47–63
Whitehead M, Godfree V 1992 Hormone replacement therapy: your questions answered. Churchill Livingstone, Edinburgh, Ch 4

MENOPAUSE

The word '**menopause**' refers to a woman's last menstrual period and marks the end of reproductive life. The term '**climacteric**' describes the years of decreasing ovarian function that has an effect on bones, blood vessels and collagen. Common terms around the menopause are shown in Box 6.2.

The average age when the menopause occurs is 51 years, the range being 45–55 years. Menopause before the age of 45 years is described as premature. Premature menopause can occur in 1% of women before the age of 40 (Chamberlain 1995). Women who smoke have their menopause about two years earlier than non-smokers (Coope 1997).

Women who have had a hysterectomy, with conservation of their ovaries, will experience the symptoms of ovarian failure earlier than otherwise.

Box 6.2 Common terms around the menopause

- **Menopause** – permanent cessation of menstruation resulting from the loss of ovarian follicular activity.
- **Climacteric** or **perimenopause** – the transitional phase leading up to the menopause and continuing for at least the first 12 months after the menopause, usually lasting for 2–3 years.
- **Postmenopause** – the state following 12 months of amenorrhoea; the life expectancy of a woman reaching the menopause is 81 years: thus a woman can expect to spend one-third of her life in the postmenopause (Payne 1997).

Age at menopause appears to be unaffected by (Abernethy 1997):

- race
- use of oral contraception
- number of pregnancies
- age of menarche
- socio-economic factors.

The menopause occurs because:

- the ovaries run out of primordial follicles
- the ovary becomes less and less responsive to the effects of follicle-stimulating hormone (FSH)

- production of oestrogen declines
- pituitary production of FSH rises due to negative feedback mechanism
- more frequent anovulation leads to loss of progesterone production by the ovary
- oestrogen production falls below a critical level, no longer stimulating the endometrium.

Menopause may be:

- natural
- surgical
- premature
- iatrogenic (following chemotherapy, radiotherapy or other drug therapy).

Menstruation prior to the menopause may be:

- irregular
- less frequent
- more frequent
- less heavy or scanty
- occasionally very heavy
- irregular, then revert to previous pattern
- rarely, quite regular until it suddenly stops.

NB The timescale for changes is extremely variable and can differ greatly from woman to woman. The climacteric and post-menopause are states of oestrogen deficiency. Oestrogen deficiency has short-, intermediate- and long-term consequences.

Nursing issues

Spend some time thinking about the following:

- accurate information about the physiological and psychological events during the climacteric and beyond
- promoting a healthy lifestyle
- identifying those women at particular risk of the consequences of oestrogen deficiency
- providing current information about the risks/benefits of various therapies, including HRT and alternative therapies
- respecting the individual beliefs of those asking for information
- assisting access to appropriate therapies
- providing information about local and national resources and groups.

SYMPTOMS OF THE MENOPAUSE

Short- and intermediate-term symptoms typically attributed to the menopause are as follows:

Short-term symptoms

Vasomotor symptoms:

- hot flushes
- night sweats
- palpitations
- headaches.

Menstrual disturbances:

- irregular, prolonged or heavy periods.

Psychological symptoms:

- insomnia
- mood swings
- poor concentration
- anxiety
- fatigue
- poor memory
- sexual difficulties/anxieties
- depression.

Short-term (climacteric) symptoms are self-limiting and gradually subside as the levels of circulating oestrogen stop fluctuating and fall to a low, steady level (Payne 1997).

Intermediate symptoms

Intermediate symptoms affecting epithelial and connective tissues:

- vaginal dryness
- vulval and vaginal atrophy
- dyspareunia
- vaginitis
- bladder dysfunction/urethral syndrome
- uterovaginal prolapse
- thinning of skin and hair
- joint and muscle pain.

Long-term effects

Long-term effects of oestrogen deficiency are osteoporosis and cardiovascular disease.

Severity and extent of menopausal symptoms

Seventy to 80% of women experience some oestrogen-deficiency symptoms, with hot flushes being the most common. There is little or no correlation between plasma oestradiol levels and incidence or severity of symptoms.

Symptoms experienced are described as mild in 16% of women, moderate in 33% and severe in 51%. Twenty-five per cent of women have symptoms for 5 years (Abernethy 1997).

The prevalence of symptoms varies between cultures. For example, only 20% of Japanese women experience hot flushes. There is no firm explanation for this but it may be because of a higher level of 'natural' dietary oestrogen, also called phytoestrogens (see p 190).

Depression and other psychological symptoms are frequently attributed to the menopause; however, there is no compelling evidence that the hormonal changes at the climacteric cause depression in women. From Coope's 1996 review of the literature some conclusions can be made:

- Depression is common in middle-aged women.
- Depressive illness is no commoner at the menopause.
- Only flushes, night sweats and vaginal dryness are proven to be associated with ovarian failure.
- Symptoms of anxiety and depression are more likely to be due to psychosocial causes.

Whitehead & Godfree (1992) conclude that significant decreases in psychological complaints, such as irritability, fatigue, anxiety and depression are found when HRT is given.

The menopause is a natural event, it is not an illness, and there is help available to deal with some of the changes occurring at this time of life. There are many different life events that coincide with the menopause. Some women will experience only a few of these events, others will experience many. Some of these events include:

- children growing up and leaving home
- marital/relationship difficulties

- divorce
- family illness
- ageing parents
- bereavement
- accepting growing older
- adjusting to own/partner's employment changes
- accepting the end of fertility.

For many women the menopause is a very positive experience:

- no more periods, and associated problems
- no further risk of pregnancy
- fewer responsibilities
- greater self-confidence
- in some cultures post-menopausal women have higher social status.

DIAGNOSING THE MENOPAUSE

If a woman is in her 40s or early 50s diagnosis can be made by symptoms and history alone. However, menopausal symptoms may be confused with the following conditions:

- pregnancy
- dysfunctional uterine bleeding
- thyroid or adrenal disorder
- exercise-induced amenorrhoea.

Measurement of FSH can be useful when:

- premature menopause is suspected
- the woman has had a hysterectomy.

An FSH above 30 iu/l is diagnostic of ovarian failure.

Pregnancy in women over 45 years carries high risk of:

- miscarriage
- maternal and perinatal mortality
- congenital abnormality.

CONTRACEPTION

Women can ovulate up to the menopause. Six months of amenorrhoea can be followed by ovulation. A woman who has her last menstrual period before 50 years should use contraception for two years. A woman who has her last menstrual period after 50 years should use contraception for one year. HRT is not a contraceptive.

Methods used, according to the woman's wishes and lifestyle, may include:

- combined oral contraceptive (as long as there are no cardiovascular contraindications and the woman understands the risks)
- progestogen-only pill (amenorrhoea with this pill may be confused with the menopause)
- injectable progestogens (can cause amenorrhoea or irregular bleeding)
- barriers (diaphragm or condoms)
- IUD or IUS (copper or levonorgestrel-bearing intrauterine device or system)
- natural methods (difficult to carry out, unpredictable cycles making them unreliable).

MENOPAUSE AND CARDIOVASCULAR DISEASE

Cardiovascular disease is the most common cause of death among women in the UK. Non-smoking premenopausal women rarely suffer heart attacks and strokes. By the time a woman is 70, however, she has the same cardiovascular risks as a man. In addition, postmenopausal women who have a myocardial infarction (MI) have almost double the mortality of a man of the same age (possibly due to underestimation of symptoms and delay in diagnosis; Payne 1997). Women are:

- more likely to die within 60 days of an MI
- 45% die within a year of an MI
- more likely to have a second MI (Payne 1997).

Women tend to have more severe coronary heart disease (CHD) at presentation than men, more severe MIs than men and a worse prognosis than men. Women with CHD tend to have lower rates of diagnostic tests and treatment procedures than men (Sharp 1998).

Oestrogen appears to be cardioprotective by probably:

- reducing LDL
- increasing high-density lipoprotein (HDL)

- causing dilatation of coronary arteries
- affecting the tone of arteries, possibly influencing blood pressure (Whitehead & Godfree 1992).

The management of some menopausal symptoms and difficulties is shown in Box 6.3.

Box 6.3 Management of menopausal symptoms

Problem	Possible solution	Effect
Lifestyle	Stop smoking	Decreases cardiovascular and osteoporosis risk
	Achieve good diet	Optimum calcium intake (see p 199) maintains health of bone; 'naturally' occurring oestrogens (e.g. in soya, yam, red clover) may reduce flushes, etc.
	Increase exercise	Maintains bone mass; improves well-being; aids relaxation
	Weight control	Improves well-being; obesity increases cardiovascular risks
	Limit alcohol consumption	Affects calcium absorption; increases hot flushes; excess increases cardiovascular risks
Hot flushes/night sweats	Use natural fibres for clothes and bed linen; keep a cool environment; limit certain drinks and foods	Fewer flushes/sweats
	Gamolenic acid, starflower oil, vitamin E	May relieve flushes/sweats
	Clonidine (antihypertensive)	Fewer flushes/sweats
	HRT	No flushes/sweats
Vaginal dryness	Rehydration creams/gels	May relieve temporarily
	Oestrogen cream	Can greatly relieve
	HRT	Can greatly relieve
Osteoporosis risk	Healthy lifestyle/diet	Reduces risk
	HRT	Prevents bone loss
Cardiovascular disease risk	Healthy lifestyle/diet	Reduces risk
	HRT	Reduces risk
Psychological symptoms	Yoga, meditation, reflexology, acupuncture, etc.	May reduce stress, improve well-being

Box 6.3	Management of menopausal symptoms (*Continued*)	
Problem	*Possible solution*	*Effect*
	Aromatherapy, homeopathy, etc.	May reduce stress, improve well-being
	HRT	Can improve well-being, possibly decreases risk of Alzheimer's disease (see p. 177)

Key points

- A woman who has had a premature menopause has a two-fold increase in cardiovascular disease risk.
- Any vaginal bleeding after the menopause *must* be investigated.
- Any woman who is seeking information about the menopause should be able to take advantage of the following procedures:
  - weight monitoring
  - blood pressure measurement
  - serum cholesterol measurement (depending on family history)
  - bone density scan (if indicated)
  - cervical smear (if due)
  - mammogram (if due)
  - education about becoming breast-aware.
- The RCN (1997) have published guidance on management of the menopause.

REFERENCES

Abernethy K 1997 The menopause and hormone replacement therapy. Baillière Tindall, London, Ch 1

Chamberlain G (ed) 1995 Gynaecology by ten teachers, 16th edn. Arnold, London, Ch 1

Coope J 1996 Hormonal and non-hormonal interventions for menopausal women. Maturitas 23: 159–168

Coope J 1997 The menopause. In: McPherson A, Waller D (eds) Women's health, 4th edn. Oxford University Press, Oxford, Ch 11

Payne E 1997 Menopausal problems. In: Luesley D (ed) Common conditions in gynaecology. Chapman & Hall, London, Ch 13

RCN 1997 The menopause, osteoporosis and hormone replacement therapy: an RCN guide for nurses, midwives and health visitors. Royal College of Nursing, London

Sharp I 1998 Gender issues in the prevention and treatment of coronary heart disease. In: Doyal L (ed) Women and health services. Open University Press, Buckingham, Ch 6

Whitehead M, Godfree V 1992 Hormone replacement therapy: your questions answered. Churchill Livingstone, Edinburgh, Ch 4

FURTHER READING

Abernethy K 1997 The menopause and HRT. Baillière Tindall, London
Coope J 1997 The menopause. In: McPherson A, Waller D (eds) Women's health, 4th edn. Oxford University Press, Oxford, Ch 11
Niven C, Walker A (eds) 1996 Reproductive potential and fertility control. Butterworth-Heinemann, Oxford

RESOURCES

British Menopause Society, 36 West Street, Marlow S07 2NB, UK. Tel.: 01628 890199.
Family Planning Association, 2–12 Pentonville Road, London N1 9FP, UK (booklet).
National Osteoporosis Society, PO Box 10, Radstock, Bath BA3 3YB, UK. Tel: 01761 432472.
The Amarant Trust, 11–13 Charterhouse Buildings, London EC1M 7AN, UK. Tel: 01293 413000 (helpline).
Women's Health Concern, PO Box 1629, London SW15 2ZL, UK. Tel: 020 8780 3916 (helpline).
Women's Health Information Service, 52–54 Featherstone Street, London EC1Y 8RT (information).

OSTEOPOROSIS

Osteoporosis is a disease characterized by:

- low bone mass
- disruption of bone architecture
- reduced bone strength
- increased risk of fracture.

Osteoporosis may be:

- primary or age-related
- secondary to disease or drugs.

Osteoporosis itself is painless; osteoporotic fractures can be extremely painful and limit activities of daily living.

WHY IS OSTEOPOROSIS A PROBLEM?

Osteoporosis affects one in four women. The estimated number of osteoporotic fractures in UK each year are 60 000 of hip, 50 000 of radius and 40 000 of vertebrae (NOS 1996). By the age of 70 years 50% of women will have had at least one osteoporotic fracture (Chamberlain 1995). About 28% of women who have a hip fracture die as a direct result (Payne 1997).

The estimated cost of osteoporotic fractures in England and Wales is £742 million (Compston et al 1995).

NORMAL BONE AND PEAK BONE MASS

Normal, healthy bone is maintained through a balance of bone-building osteoblasts and bone resorption by osteoclastic activity. Normal nutrition and growth lead to a peak bone mass by the mid-30s. The absorption and availability of calcium is affected by vitamin D, while calcium regulation is influenced by calcitonin (a thyroid hormone) and parathormone (a parathyroid hormone).

Peak bone mass is largely genetically determined, but it may be reduced by poor nutrition or illness in childhood. After achieving peak bone mass, around the mid-30s, bone is lost at 1% a year until approaching the menopause. Bone loss accelerates to 3–5% a year around the menopause and for up to 10 years after (NOS 1996).

Oestrogen deficiency affects the rate of bone loss. A woman will have lost almost 50% of her bone mass by the age of 70.

Nursing opportunities to provide health education and the promotion of a lifestyle to prevent osteoporosis are many, e.g. by:

- midwife
- health visitor
- school nurse
- practice nurse

Nursing issues

Spend some time thinking about the following:

- encouraging all patients to adopt a lifestyle which will enable them to reach and sustain a high peak bone mass
- identifying those at risk of osteoporosis, e.g.
  - on long-term steroid usage
  - premature menopause
  - previous fracture
  - hysterectomized women
- encouraging those at risk to have hormone replacement therapy (HRT)
- ensuring that those with established osteoporosis are receiving appropriate treatment to prevent further bone loss
- ensuring that there is adequate pain relief
- enabling patients to maintain optimum levels of function and independence.

- occupational health nurse
- district nurse
- family planning nurse.

RISK FACTORS

Factors significantly increasing the risk of osteoporosis are shown in Box 6.4.

Box 6.4 Risk factors for osteoporosis (NOS/RCN 1996)	
General	• premature menopause (before age 45)
	• secondary oestrogen deficiency in anorexia nervosa
	• female athlete over-exercise syndrome
	• hyperprolactinaemia and other causes of primary and secondary amenorrhoea
Medical problems	• high dose or long-term steroid usage
	• Cushing's syndrome
	• previous low-impact trauma fractures
	• immobilizing diseases
	• chronic liver disease or malabsorption
	• hyperthyroidism and over-treatment with thyroxine
	• gastrectomy
Genetic	• strong family history
Lifestyle	• excessive alcohol consumption
	• smoking
	• low calcium intake

Other factors

Other factors are:

- Little exposure to daylight.
- Racial origin (black women have higher levels of calcitonin and higher peak bone mass than white women) (Whitehead & Godfree 1992).
- Low body mass (young women with anorexia nervosa are unlikely to reach their potential peak bone density) (Waller 1997).

Calcium

There is no consensus about the role of dietary calcium. Some opinions:

- An increase of milk consumption in adolescent girls can enhance bone mineral acquisition (Barker et al 1997).
- Dietary calcium does not influence either post-menopausal bone loss or its response to therapy (Stevenson 1992).
- The efficiency of calcium absorption from the gut decreases with age.
- Excessive alcohol consumption inhibits the absorption of calcium.

PREVENTION

Prevention is either through lifestyle or is therapeutic.

Box 6.5 Lifestyle factors in osteoporosis prevention	
Healthy diet	to ensure intake of calcium rich foods is adequate (see p. 199)
Smoking	suppresses osteoclast activity, affects oestrogen metabolism, smokers tend to have lower body weight
Alcohol	excess reduces calcium absorption, damages liver and bone cells
Exercise	regular weight-bearing exercise can increase bone formation (brisk walking, keep fit, dancing); exercise must be maintained
Fall prevention	limit opportunities for falls

Lifestyle

Lifestyle factors in osteoporosis prevention are shown in Box 6.5.

Therapeutic prevention

There are therapies that can prevent bone loss and fractures (Box 6.6). The incidence of osteoporosis is greater in women than in men (10:1). This is because oestrogen deficiency after the

Box 6.6 Recommended minimum daily doses of different oestrogens to prevent osteoporosis	
Conjugated oestrogens	0.625 mg
Oral oestradiol	2 mg
Transdermal oestradiol	50 mg
Oestradiol valerate	2 mg
Tibolone	2.5 mg

menopause results in a rapid loss of bone density. Replacing oestrogen in the form of HRT (see p. 176) will prevent bone loss and maintain bone density.

Starting HRT near the menopause and taking it for a minimum of 5 years reduces the incidence of hip fractures by 50% (Abernethy 1997). Women who have had a premature menopause (spontaneously or as a result of surgery, radiotherapy or chemotherapy) should be strongly encouraged to take HRT to prevent osteoporosis and cardiovascular disease in the future (see p. 200).

The Primary Care Rheumatology Society (1997) (a consensus group of general practitioners and hospital specialists) has produced guidelines to clarify the strength of any recommendation for treatment (Box 6.7; these guidelines are under review and will be updated).

Box 6.7 Guidelines produced by the Primary Care Rheumatology Group (1997)

Absolute recommendation	*Strong recommendation*	*Possible recommendation*
• Early menopause • Use of corticosteroids • Multiple atraumatic fractures • Anorexia nervosa	• History of late menarche • Secondary amenorrhoea • Chronic liver disease • History of prolonged bed-rest	• Osteoporosis in primary relatives • Heavy smokers • High alcohol intake • Women concerned about osteoporosis

---

DIAGNOSIS

Diagnosis of osteoporosis is by:

- accurate history
- exclude other coexisting disease
- X-ray gives limited information
  - 30% of bone mass must be lost before changes are picked up on X-ray
  - can demonstrate vertebral crush fractures
  - is too insensitive to monitor response to treatment.

Bone densitometry

The following techniques provide a direct measurement of bone mass:

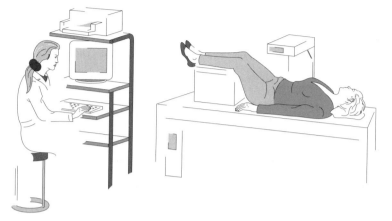

Figure 6.1   Bone densitometer. Research is ongoing to develop a machine to measure bone density through the heel.

- single photon absorptiometry (SPA)
- dual photon absorptiometry (DPA)
- quantitative computerized tomography (QCT)
- dual energy X-ray absorptiometry (DEXA), which provides the most accurate means of measuring bone mass and so predicting osteoporosis risk before fractures occur (see Fig. 6.1). Unfortunately it is not readily available.

Fracture risk is directly related to bone density.

The Primary Care Rheumatology Society has guidelines for management following bone density scanning (Box 6.8).

Box 6.8   Guidelines for management following bone scanning

Normal bone mass with no fracture	Bone mass 1.5–2.5 standard deviations below mean	Low bone mass i.e. >2.5 standard deviations below mean	Fracture
↓	↓	↓	↓
No treatment	Assess and monitor the individual and repeat scan in 1 year	Treat with HRT or cyclical etidronate if vertebral fracture already present	Treat with HRT or cyclical etidronate if vertebral fracture already present, or refer to specialist unit

---

TREATMENT

Treatment of established osteoporosis is by use of antiresorptive agents, which decrease bone resorption, and some produce a

Box 6.9 Treatment of osteoporosis		
Bisphosphonates	Slow down osteoclast activity	• alendronic acid (oral) • disodium etidronate (oral)
Calcium	May reduce rate of bone loss	• 800 mg daily (larger doses are not more effective) (BNF)
	Low levels of vitamin D can reduce calcium absorption (e.g. in housebound)	• vitamin D 400 iu daily, usually combined with a calcium supplement (e.g. Calcichew) (oral)
Vitamin D metabolites	Increase calcium absorption	• calcitriol (oral)
Calcitonin	Reduces osteoclast activity	• Salcatonin (s.c. or i.m. injection)

significant increase in bone mass, which is associated with a reduction in the rate of vertebral or hip fractures (NOS/RCN 1996). Treatments are:

- oestrogens
- bisphosphonates
- calcium supplements, with or without vitamin D
- vitamin D metabolites
- calcitonin.

(Box 6.9)

Other agents stimulate bone formation, however they have considerable side-effects and currently are not licensed for the treatment of osteoporosis, e.g.:

- anabolic steroids
- sodium fluoride
- parathyroid hormone.

SERMs appear to have all the benefits of oestrogen with few of the disadvantages. One (raloxifene) is undergoing extensive trials, having so far shown it can significantly increase bone mineral density in lumbar spine, hip and whole skeleton (Delmas et al 1997).

Once osteoporosis is established it is important to ensure the following:

- optimum, appropriate treatment
- monitoring the effect of treatment
- encouragement of a healthy lifestyle

- physiotherapy
- adequate pain relief
- contact with local and national organizations for support and information.

Dietary calcium is available from a wide variety of foods, e.g.:

- dairy produce (milk, cheese, yoghurt)
- green vegetables (spinach, broccoli, winter cabbage, spring greens)
- tinned fish (salmon, sardines, pilchards)
- nuts (brazil nuts, hazelnuts, peanuts)
- dried fruits (figs, apricots)
- beans (baked beans, kidney beans)
- ice cream
- milk chocolate and various chocolate bars.

The National Osteoporosis Society (NOS) recommends a daily intake of dietary calcium, that will vary throughout life (Table 6.1).

Table 6.1 Lifetime intake of dietary calcium

Age group	Daily calcium intake
Children 7–12 years	800 mg
Teenagers 13–19 years	1000 mg
Women 20–45 years	1000 mg
Pregnant and nursing teenagers	1500 mg
Pregnant and nursing women	1200 mg
Women over 45 years	1500 mg
Women over 45 years taking HRT	1000 mg

Key points

- The first sign that a woman has osteoporosis may be:
  - loss of height
  - the severe pain caused by osteoporotic fractures.
- Be aware of any woman who has sustained a bone fracture with the minimum of trauma: e.g. woman of 45 who suffers an ankle fracture from a minor slip.
- Carrying out a bone density scan on a woman who was previously unaware of her risk of osteoporosis can help her to modify her risk factors and consider therapeutic interventions.

REFERENCES

Abernethy K 1997 The menopause and HRT. Baillière Tindall, London
Barker M, Cadogan J, Eastell R 1997 Milk intake and bone mineral acquisition in adolescent girls: randomised, controlled intervention trial. British Medical Journal 315: 1255–1260
Chamberlain G 1995 (ed) Gynaecology by ten teachers, 16th edn. Arnold, London, Ch 1
Compston J, Cooper C, Kanis J 1995 Bone densitometry in clinical practice. British Medical Journal 310: 1308–1310
Delmas M, Bjarnason N, Mitlak B et al 1997 Effects of raloxifene on bone mineral density, serum cholesterol concentrations and uterine endometrium in post menopausal women. New England Journal of Medicine 337: 1641–1647
NOS 1996 Have you broken a bone? National Osteoporosis Society
NOS/RCN 1996 Osteoporosis Resource Pack: For nurses, midwives and health visitors. National Osteoporosis Society/Royal College of Nursing
Payne E 1997 Menopausal problems. In: Luesley D (ed) Common conditions in gynaecology. Chapman & Hall, London, Ch 13
Primary Care Rheumatology Society 1997 Osteoporosis: primary care consensus guidelines on diagnosis and treatment. Cited in 'Guidelines'. Primary Care Rheumatology Society, Northallerton
Stevenson J 1992 Prevention and treatment of osteoporosis. Women's Health Concern, London
Waller D 1997 Eating disorders. In: McPherson A, Waller D (eds) Women's health, 4th edn. Oxford University Press, Oxford, Ch 18

FURTHER READING

Abernethy K 1997 The menopause and HRT. Baillière Tindall, London
Coope J 1997 The menopause. In: McPherson A, Waller D (eds) Women's health, 4th edn. Oxford University Press, Oxford, Ch 11

RESOURCES

National Osteoporosis Society, PO Box 10, Radstock, Bath BA3 3YB, Tel.: 01761 471771 (information, leaflets and resource pack).

WOMEN AND CARDIOVASCULAR DISEASE

Cardiovascular disease includes coronary heart disease (CHD)/ischaemic heart disease and hypertension. It can lead to heart attacks and strokes. It is highly significant as the leading cause of death in women, with one in four women dying from cardiovascular disease. Until recently cardiovascular disease risk was considered a male problem, with all research and interventions directed at men (Sharp 1998). Awareness among health professionals and the public is now rising.

Nursing issues

Spend some time thinking about the following:

- awareness of the morbidity and mortality of cardiovascular disease in women
- identification of those with additional risk factors
- promotion of a healthy lifestyle
- enabling those at risk to modify or change lifestyle
- understanding social, cultural and racial influences on lifestyle and risk factors
- knowledge of therapeutic interventions
- demonstrating sensitivity when dealing with individual beliefs and anxieties.

RISK FACTORS

These may be classified into three groups: fixed factors, which cannot be modified; strongly associated factors, which can be modified by change or treatment; and weakly associated factors, which have not been proven or disproven to affect risks.

Fixed factors

Fixed factors are:

- age (risks increase with age)
- positive family history
- possible genetic predisposition.

Strongly associated factors

Strongly associated factors are:

- Hyperlipidaemia – raised plasma cholesterol levels are associated with a high risk of atherosclerosis and increased risk of CHD, the level of risk rising with the increased level of cholesterol; if following a low-cholesterol diet does not reduce high levels, then cholesterol-lowering drugs should be used.
- Cigarette smoking – smoking increases and exacerbates atherosclerosis and thrombus formation; all stopping-smoking measures should be encouraged.

- Hypertension – complications of hypertension include stroke, ischaemic heart disease and heart failure; treatment of hypertension is effective if carried out according to current guidelines.
- Diabetes mellitus – ischaemic heart disease is the major cause of mortality among diabetics and diabetes is a significant risk factor for coronary artery disease; awareness of these risks and addressing other risk factors is essential.
- Exercise – lack of exercise increases the risk of coronary artery disease, and regular exercise probably protects against its development (Camm 1994).

Weakly associated factors

Weakly associated factors are:

- Personality – the 'type A' personality that is characterized by unsuccessful aggression, ambition, compulsion and competitiveness is said to be more frequently associated with CHD.
- Obesity – it is uncertain if obesity is an independent risk factor, however it is likely to be linked to poor diet and lack of exercise (Camm 1994).
- Heavy alcohol consumption – it appears that moderate levels of alcohol have a protective effect against CHD, but heavy consumption may increase atherosclerosis.
- Contraceptive pill – the combined oral contraceptive pill increases the risk of heart attack and stroke, particularly in women aged over 35 who are smokers (Guillebaud 1997).

Non-smoking, premenopausal women rarely suffer from heart attacks or strokes. However, by 10 years after the menopause, women have the same incidence of heart attack as men.

Changes in lipid profile may be responsible for:

- lowering HDL
- raising LDL
- increasing total cholesterol.

These changes in lipid profile are atherogenic, producing atheromatous plaques in arteries. There are also possible changes in platelet function, together with a possible decrease in peripheral blood flow (Chamberlain 1995).

Oestrogen appears to offer a cardioprotective effect, regardless of the age of the woman, since oestrogen:

- reduces LDL
- increases HDL
- directly affects arterial walls, increasing blood flow and decreasing blood pressure (Payne 1997).

Extensive trials of oestrogen replacement have demonstrated significant reduction in cardiovascular events in women, potentially leading to up to 40% reduction in heart attacks and up to 20% reduction in strokes.

SMOKING AND CORONARY HEART DISEASE (CHD) (White 1993)

- Cigarette smokers are twice as likely to die of CHD as never-smokers.
- Smoking may account for two-thirds of myocardial infarctions (MI) in women under 50.
- Stopping smoking halves the additional risk of CHD after one year of stopping.
- Fifteen years after stopping the risk is the same as for a never-smoker.
- After one MI stopping smoking significantly reduces risk of further MI.
- Smokers, over 35 years, who take the combined pill have a tenfold risk of a cardiovascular event.

(White 1993)

HYPERTENSION

The British Hypertension Society (1998) has published general recommendations on the management of hypertension. These state: 'It remains an issue of much concern that around half of treated hypertensive patients do not achieve acceptable blood pressure control'. Treatment goals are as follows:

- diastolic blood pressure (DBP) to be < 90 mmHg
- systolic blood pressure (SBP) – no firm recommendations can be made but it is considered prudent to reduce SBP to at least <160 mmHg.

Recommendations

- Use non-pharmological (i.e. lifestyle modification) measures in all people who are hypertensive.
- In addition, initiate drug treatment in patients with sustained DBP >100 mmHg.
- Decide on treatment in patients with sustained DBP between 90 and 99 mmHg according to the presence of target organ damage and/or other risk factors (e.g. heart failure or renal disease).
- Treat elderly patients with SBP >160 mmHg and/or DBP > 90 mmHg.
- Currently recommended are either diuretics or beta blockers as first line therapy. However, where these are contraindicated, ineffective, or, when side-effects occur, or in selected conditions, there may be a role for newer agents, as first line therapy. These agents include angiotension-converting enzyme (ACE) inhibitors, calcium channel blockers and alpha blockers.

REFERENCES

British Hypertension Society 1998. Management guidelines in essential hypertension. Heart 80 (Suppl 2): 21–29

Camm AJ 1994 Cardiovascular disease. In: Kumar P, Clark M (eds) Clinical medicine, 3rd edn. Saunders, London, Ch 11

Chamberlain G (ed) 1995 Gynaecology by ten teachers, 16th edn. Arnold, London, Ch 1

Guillebaud J 1997 The pill. Oxford University Press, Oxford

Payne E 1997 Menopausal problems. In: Luesley D (ed) Common conditions in gynaecology. Chapman & Hall, London, Ch 13

Sharp I 1998 Gender issues in the prevention and treatment of coronary heart disease. In: Doyal L (ed) Women and health services. Open University Press, Buckingham, Ch 6

White P 1993 Women and smoking. In: McPherson A (ed) Women's problems in general practice, 3rd edn. Oxford University Press, Oxford, Ch 19

7

Sensitive issues

This chapter explores some of the issues that may be sensitive, both for the woman and for the nurse who is caring for her.

ABORTION

Abortion is the deliberate termination of a pregnancy. The Abortion Act 1967 legalized termination of pregnancy, and was amended by the Human Fertilisation and Embryology Act in 1990.

The legal requirement: two registered medical practitioners must agree that the criteria have been met:

that the pregnancy has not exceeded 24 weeks and that the continuation of the pregnancy would involve risk, greater than if the pregnancy were terminated, or injury to the physical or mental health of the pregnant woman or any existing children of her family.

In extreme circumstances there is no time limit to termination of pregnancy. These include the risk:

• of grave permanent injury to the mother
• to the life of the mother
• of serious fetal abnormality.

Fetal reduction (the termination of one or more, but not all fetuses) can be considered in multiple pregnancy.

All clinics offering abortion have to be approved and regulated by the Department of Health. Abortions after 24 weeks have to be carried out in NHS hospitals. Health authorities are not legally required to provide an abortion service.

The Abortion Act (1967) does not apply in Northern Ireland, where an abortion can only be carried out very rarely and in exceptional circumstances.

There is a 'conscience clause' in the Abortion Act (1967): someone who has very strong beliefs may refuse to participate in an abortion procedure. Exceptional situations are excluded from the conscience clause, for example, where a woman may bleed to death if she does not have an abortion. Conscientious objection does not extend to those who are remotely connected to the abortion process, for example, the secretary to the gynaecologist (McHale 1998).

Information given to any woman contemplating an abortion should include (RCN 1996):

• the choices available to her
• the procedures involved
• the investigations that may be required (e.g. post-mortem)
• her future fertility and pregnancies
• contraceptive choices
• genetic counselling, if appropriate
• details of relevant support groups.

Nursing issues

Spend some time thinking about the following:

- recognition that all women have a right to
  - information, choice and support
  - an accessible, confidential service
  - non-judgmental care provided by competently trained staff
- consideration to be given to the individual, religious and cultural needs of each woman
- awareness of the sensitive and difficult issues for each woman
- awareness of one's own beliefs and prejudices
- awareness of the moral and ethical issues involved
- ensuring the woman has access to appropriate care when there are difficulties of conscience
- awareness of the inequalities of abortion provision throughout the country
- knowledge of local and national services and resources.

GUIDELINES

Nurses and Abortion. Issues in nursing and health. No 11. Royal College of Nursing, 1992
Fetal Cell Transplantation: Guidance For Nurses. Issues in nursing and health. No 7. Royal College of Nursing, 1994
Guidelines on the Termination of Pregnancy. Royal College of Nursing, 1997.

UNINTENDED PREGNANCY

Up to 50% of all pregnancies may be unplanned.
The woman's options are:

- Continue with the pregnancy and have the baby.
- Continue with the pregnancy and have the baby adopted (giving information as to how to access adoption services).
- Terminate the pregnancy.

Counselling must be available to any woman contemplating an abortion – the extent of the counselling depending on each woman's needs and situation (Davidson 1997, Gray 1997).

In England and Wales in 1994 20% of all recorded pregnancies were terminated, 53% of pregnancies in the under 16 s were terminated and 40% of pregnancies in the over 40s were terminated (Office for National Statistics 1996). Table 7.1 shows abortion statistics for 1994.

Some reasons for unplanned pregnancy:

- inadequate sex education
- ignorance
- lack of knowledge of contraceptive services and how to access them
- lack of awareness of emergency contraception
- coercion
- rape
- risk-taking
- low self-esteem (not feeling you are worth looking after; grateful for any attention)
- contraceptive failure
- believing self to be infertile.

Every woman has her own unique set of circumstances. Some wanted pregnancies become unwanted. Some unwanted pregnancies end up being very wanted.

Table 7.1 Abortion statistics for 1994 by age group

Age group	Abortion rates per 1000 women
Under 15	3.4
15	7.1
16–19	22.0
20–24	25.4
25–29	18.6
30–34	12.6
35–39	8.0
40–44	3.0
45 and over	0.2
All ages	12.2

Source: Office for National Statistics 1996

METHODS OF ABORTION

Abortion may be carried out by either surgical or medical techniques. Eighty-five to 90% of abortions are carried out in the first 12 weeks of gestation.

Surgical techniques

- Suction or vacuum termination:
  - up to 12 weeks' gestation using general anaesthetic
  - up to 9 weeks' gestation using local anaesthetic

- usually carried out as day case.
- Dilatation and evacuation (D&E):
  - can be used from 13–20 weeks
  - usually only used up to 16 weeks
  - under general anaesthetic.

Medical techniques

- Early medical abortion:
  - up to 9 weeks' gestation
  - using mifepristone, a progesterone antagonist (progesterone is essential for maintaining a pregnancy)
  - no anaesthetic, but analgesia as required
  - 3 tablets orally followed by a vaginal pessary 48 hours later
  - carried out in a dedicated unit
  - 95% will abort within 6 hours of the pessary
  - up to 5% will require a surgical procedure, either not having aborted or having aborted incompletely
  - not suitable for smokers aged over 35 (it would increase the risk of thrombosis).
- Late medical abortion:
  - using prostaglandins to stimulate uterine contractions and induce labour
  - mifepristone may be given 48 hours before prostaglandins
  - involves a stay in hospital
  - takes an average of 12 hours
  - can be very painful and distressing
  - will need surgical procedure if the placenta is retained.

Risks

The risks include:

- risks of any anaesthetic
- perforation of uterus (1 in 500)
- damage to cervix (possible stenosis or incompetence)
- pelvic infection (less likely with sexually transmitted infection screening prior to procedure)
- haemorrhage.

Death may occur, with an incidence of about 1 in 100 000 abortions, usually due to haemorrhage, infection, pulmonary embolus or anaesthetic complications (Afnan & Mann 1997).

Some women feel regret following abortion. This may be for a number of reasons:

- for having had to make the choice
- for having failed to prevent the pregnancy in the first place
- for having the abortion
- for the baby that never was
- for the lack of a relationship that would support a pregnancy
- for having a genetic disorder or a baby with a congenital abnormality.

Regret and depression are more likely following a late therapeutic abortion. Ambivalence about the decision or any element of coercion to have an abortion are more likely to result in depression. Most women who choose to have an abortion and who have been appropriately supported and counselled in their decision feel little other than relief. Choosing to have an abortion is significant decision made at a time of crisis (Walker 1996, Davidson 1997, Gray 1997).

REFERENCES

Afnan M, Mann M 1997 Fertility control. In: Luesley D (ed) Common conditions in gynaecology. Chapman & Hall, London, Ch 8

Davidson L 1997 Unwanted pregnancy and abortion. In: McPherson A, Waller D (eds) Women's health, 4th edn. Oxford University Press, Oxford, Ch 7

Gray K 1997 Unplanned pregnancy. In: Andrews G (ed) Women's sexual health. Baillière Tindall, London, Ch 7

McHale J 1998 Reproductive choice. In: McHale J, Tingle J, Peysner J (eds) Law and nursing. Butterworth Heinemann, Oxford, Ch 11

Office for National Statistics 1996. Abortion statistics 1994. HMSO, London

RCN 1996 Nurses and abortion. Issues in nursing and health 11. Royal College of Nursing, London

Walker A 1996 Psychological aspects of elective abortion. In: Niven C, Walker A (eds) Reproductive potential and fertility control. Butterworth Heinemann, Oxford, Ch 9

FURTHER READING

Baird D 1995 Therapeutic abortion. In: Loudon N, Glasier A, Gebbie A (eds) Handbook of family planning and reproductive health care, 3rd edn. Churchill Livingstone, Edinburgh, Ch 10

McHale J 1998 Reproductive choice. In: McHale J, Tingle J, Peysner J (eds) Law and nursing. Butterworth-Heinemann, Oxford, Ch 11

DOMESTIC VIOLENCE

Domestic violence may comprise physical, emotional, sexual and economic abuse occurring in an adult relationship between intimate or formerly intimate partners with a pattern of controlling behaviour by the abusing partner. Physical violence is frequently ongoing, and associated with increasing entrapment, injury, medical complaints, psychosocial problems and unsuccessful help-seeking (Richardson & Feder 1996).

Domestic violence is an extensive problem, affecting the health of women and of their children. It is vastly under-reported.

- 25% of all women are estimated to suffer some form of abuse from their partner or ex-partner.
- 25–30% of assaults reported to the police are the result of domestic violence.
- Nearly 50% of all women who are murdered are killed by their husband or partner.

Assault may start or increase during pregnancy.
The victims are more likely to:

- have poor health
- have chronic pain
- have anxiety and/or depression
- have addictions (e.g. drugs, alcohol)
- have problem pregnancies (e.g. more miscarriages, more low birthweight babies)
- attempt suicide.

There is a high risk of child abuse among the children of abused women (Richardson & Feder 1995). Domestic violence is universal, regardless of education, class, culture, economic status, race or social standing.

Signs that should make one consider it as a possibility (Heath 1994) are where:

- The extent or type of injury is inconsistent with the explanation given by the woman.
- There is a considerable delay between the time of the injury and the presentation for treatment.
- The injuries are to areas hidden by clothing (e.g. breast, chest, abdomen).

- Injuries occurring in pregnancy.
- The woman is accompanied by her partner who insists on staying close to her and answering for her.
- A history of psychiatric illness in the woman or her partner.
- A history of attempted suicide.
- A history of depression, anxiety, failure to cope, and social withdrawal, with an underlying sense of hopelessness.
- A history of behaviour problems in the children of the household.

There can be a cyclical pattern to domestic violence with three phases (Sassetti, cited by Graham-Jones and Duxbury 1997):

1. Tension-building phase:
   - the batterer makes increasingly unreasonable demands for complete obedience
   - the woman is allowed no autonomy, is constantly berated and belittled.
2. Explosive violence: the batterer behaves more and more irritably until his anger erupts.
3. Honeymoon phase:
   - the tension is defused
   - the batterer is typically doting, apologetic, and filled with remorse, until the tension begins to mount again as he strives to assert control over his partner and family.

Why do the majority of abused women fail to report incidences of physical assault to the police (Humphries 1997)?

- They did not wish to provoke their partner.
- They felt some responsibility for their injuries.
- They did not feel that the police would take them seriously.
- They were too depressed to make the decision.

Why is it so difficult for victims of domestic violence to leave their abuser?

- They have become demeaned and demoralized.
- Loss of self-esteem.
- Feeling of responsibility for their own plight.
- Fear:
  - of further violence
  - of future loneliness
  - of poverty.

- Shame.
- Previous unhelpful experience of disclosure (e.g. being offered tranquillizers by her GP).

Why it can be so difficult to consider that domestic violence has occurred (Richardson & Feder 1996):

- Too close for comfort – it is hard to think of violent behaviour in 'nice' families, professional people, 'people like us'.
- Fear of offending.
- Fear of violence from partner of woman.
- Powerlessness, to 'fix' the problem.
- Lack of time: disclosure will be too time-consuming.
- Loss of control, when interventions are useless.

What do women who are victims of domestic violence want?

- Awareness of the possibility of domestic violence.
- Recognition of signs and symptoms.

Nursing issues

- awareness of domestic violence as an issue
- awareness of the variety of settings in which a woman who is a victim of domestic violence may be seen:
  - primary care
  - Accident & Emergency
  - gynaecology
  - mental health services, for self or children
  - sexual health services
- knowledge of the importance of confidentiality
- awareness of the importance of acquiring the skills necessary to ask direct, sympathetic and non-judgemental questions
- awareness of local protocols (child protection may be an issue)
- knowledge of local and national resources and support services
- awareness of difficulty in broaching the subject and then dealing with results of a situation that may be very close to home
- awareness that, in general, abused women do not expect health care professionals to solve their problems, they want appropriate advice and information about available support services
- awareness of particular issues for women from ethnic minorities, who may not have an understanding of confidentiality and who may have communication barriers.

Key points

- Domestic violence is a taboo subject and many health professionals are reluctant to consider the possibility and broach the subject with the woman or man.

Key points (continued)

- The annual cost to the NHS of treating health problems related to domestic violence is huge, and in the Greater Glasgow area alone is estimated as £12.4 million, with a possible range of £7 million to £24 million (Monro 1998).
- Observing violence in the home of origin appears to increase the risk for men to become perpetrators and for women to become victims.
- Substance abuse, especially alcohol, by the man appears to be a significant factor (Isaac & Prothrow-Stith 1997).
- Signs can only be an *indication* of DV, *confirmation* can only come from direct questioning.
- Abused women tend to underestimate what their children have witnessed and the impact that this may have on them, particularly psychological abuse.
- 'Leaving is a process, not an act' (Monro 1998).
- It can take a very long time for a woman, demoralized by years of violence, to find the confidence and courage to choose a new life for herself and her children (Heath 1997).

- To be asked direct, sympathetic and non-judgemental questions.
- Willingness to listen and to make time.
- Appropriate advice and information about available support services.

REFERENCES

Graham-Jones S, Duxbury F 1997 Emotional disorders. In: McPherson A, Waller D (eds) Women's health, 4th edn. Oxford University Press, Oxford, Ch 17

Heath I 1994 Domestic violence and the general practitioner. Maternal and Child Health, October 316, 318, 319

Humphries L 1997 Violence at home: the prevention concept. Primary Health Care 7(1) 27–29

Isaac N, Prothrow-Stith D 1997 Violence. In: Allen KM, Phillips JM (eds) Women's health across the lifespan. Lippincott, Philadelphia, Ch 21

Monro K 1998 Domestic violence is a health service issue. RCN Women's Health Conference

Richardson J, Feder G 1995 Domestic violence against women. British Medical Journal 311: 311–312

Richardson J, Feder G 1996 Domestic violence: a hidden problem for general practice. British Journal of General Practice 46: 239–242

RESOURCES

National Domestic Violence Helpline, 0345 023 468.

National Child Protection Helpline (NSPCC), 00800 056 0566.

Refuge 24-Hour National Crisis Line, 0990 995 443.

Victim Support, 0845 30 30 900.

FEMALE GENITAL MUTILATION (FGM)

Female genital mutilation constitutes all procedures which involve partial or total removal of the external female genitalia or injury to the female genital organs whether for cultural or any other non-therapeutic reasons (WHO 1995).

TYPES OF MUTILATION

There are different types of mutilation:

- **Excision** – 85% of women and girls affected experience clitoridectomy with or without removal of the labia minora.
- **Infibulation** – 15% of women and girls experience the more radical infibulation which involves further cutting of the labia majora. The raw areas of the labia majora are then brought together to heal to form a hood over the urethra and the vagina. An artificial opening the size of a match stick is left for the passage of urine and of menstrual blood (RCN 1994).

The World Health Organization (WHO 1995) has classified four types of FGM:

- **Type I** – excision of the prepuce with or without excision of part or all of the clitoris.
- **Type II** – excision of the prepuce and clitoris together with partial or total excision of the labia minora.
- **Type III** – excision of part or all of the external genitalia and stitching/narrowing of the vaginal opening (infibulation).
- **Type IV** – unclassified: includes pricking, piercing or incision of clitoris and/or labia; cauterization by burning of clitoris and surrounding tissues; scraping of the vaginal orifice or cutting of the vagina; a number of other procedures.

Infibulation involves the removal of almost two-thirds of the female genitalia. Classification may be unhelpful, however, since mutilation varies and clitoral damage is unpredictable.

It is estimated that around the world there are between 100 and 132 million girls who have been subjected to FGM. Each year, a further 2 million girls are estimated to be at risk of the practice. Most of them live in 28 African countries, a few in the Middle East and Asian countries, and increasingly in Europe, Canada, Australia, New Zealand and the USA among immigrant communities.

The estimated prevalence is well over 80% in such countries as (WHO 1996):

- Djibouti
- Egypt
- Eritrea
- Ethiopia
- Sierra Leone
- Somalia
- Sudan.

Up to 10 000 young women are thought to be at risk of FGM in the UK (Cohen 1995).

There are no health benefits to FGM. Many reasons are given to justify the practice, including:

- custom and tradition
- religious demand
- aesthetic reasons
- protection of virginity and prevention of promiscuity.

It is important to note that FGM is not required by any religion (WHO 1995), and that the custom predates Islam. Genital surgery was performed in Europe and America to 'treat' psychosocial disorders up until the 1960s.

Female genital mutilation should be viewed as one of the extreme forms of oppression of females seen across cultures (RCN 1994).

FGM may be performed at any age from infancy to adolescence, 7 years being the average age. Although FGM is usually carried out by women, men are brought up only to want to marry a woman who has been circumcised.

The *Prohibition of Female Circumcision Act 1985* made it an offence to carry out FMG or for anyone to aid, abet, counsel or procure FGM in the UK. It is illegal to resuture a woman following delivery. Women may be de-infibulated at marriage or during pregnancy. It is possible for an infibulated woman to become pregnant without penile penetration.

HEALTH IMPLICATIONS OF FGM

Immediate

Immediate implications are:
- haemorrhage

- shock
- infection
- death.

Long-term complications

Long-term complications can include:

- problems with micturition
- recurrent urinary tract infections (largely caused by incomplete emptying of the bladder)
- vulval and dermoid cysts
- end-stage renal failure (from chronic urinary tract infection)
- menstrual problems
- chronic pelvic infection
- increased risk of vesicovaginal fistula
- sexual dysfunction
- infertility
- psychological damage.

PREGNANCY AND CHILDBIRTH
Possible complications

There are many possible complications in pregnancy and childbirth arising from FGM:

- difficulty in fetal monitoring and assessing progress of labour
- obstructed labour due to scar tissue
- severe perineal tears
- more caesarian sections
- FGM doubles the risk of mother's death in childbirth (WHO 1993)
- FGM increases the risk of the baby being born dead by three or four times (WHO 1993).

Women who have undergone FGM may be encountered in a number of settings:

- antenatal clinic
- gynaecology clinic
- family planning clinic
- Well Woman clinic
- in the community by:
  - health visitors

- school nurses
- practice nurses
- continence advisers.

Women seen in one specialist centre were likely to be in one of three situations:

- pregnant, needing full care
- non-pregnant, wanting reversal possible at marriage or for normalization
- non-pregnant, with gynaecological problems.

There are a few specialist centres dealing with FGM in this country, set up in areas where there is a need generated by a particular immigrant or refugee community.

The team comprises:

- obstetrician/gynaecologist
- specialist midwife
- skilled interpreter.

Nursing issues

Spend some time thinking about the following:

- awareness of issues of race, racism, culture and custom
- a culturally sensitive approach, avoiding labelling and stereotyping
- awareness of the particular health care needs of these women
- awareness of possible child protection issues, with some young girls being taken out of the country to have FGM performed
- knowledge of specialist services and how to access them, developing communication and networking links
- always using tact and sensitivity so that these women do not feel shame or guilt for their culture
- emphasizing confidentiality.

REFERENCES

Cohen P 1995 A painful issue. Nursing Times 91(35): 18
Prohibition of Female Circumcision Act, 1985. The Stationery Office, London
Royal College of Nursing 1994 Female genital mutilation: the unspoken issue. RCN, London
World Health Assembly 1993. Report of the World Health Organisation, 1993. World Health Organisation, Geneva
World Health Organisation 1995 Female genital mutilation. Report of a WHO Working Group 17–19 July 1995 Geneva
World Health Organisation 1996 Estimated prevalence of female genital mutilation in Africa. WHO, Geneva

FURTHER INFORMATION

Foundation for Women's Health, Research and Development (FORWARD),
40 Eastbourne Terrace, London W2 3QR, UK. Tel.: 020 7725 2606.

LESBIANISM

Lesbianism is a form of sexual variation: sexual interest or behaviour which varies from that experienced predominantly by the majority of the population (Hawton & Harrison 1997). Sexual variation is extensively underestimated – homosexuality twofold – bisexuality 13-fold (Levy 1998).

It is inappropriate to label people on the basis of their sexual preferences: for heterosexuals and homosexuals alike, sex is only one part of life (Fairburn et al 1983). However, it is valid and important in a health care context to know if a woman is a lesbian. This is because:

- it would be hard to provide good care for someone while totally ignorant of the existence of their life partner (Matthews 1998)
- information can be made appropriate and relevant to that individual, affecting subsequent treatment and care (Levy 1998).

It can be very difficult to discuss sexual preference, for any of the following reasons (Jewitt 1995):

- Assessing when it is appropriate to take a sexual history.
- Lack of confidence in discussing sex with patients.
- Fear of jeopardizing the professional–patient relationship.
- Difficulty initiating discussion of sexual health.
- Incorporating sexual health into general health.
- Embarrassment.
- Discussing sex with patients from specific religious and cultural groups.
- Language difficulties and lack of interpreters.

HEALTH ISSUES

- Lesbian women can feel excluded from the national cervical and breast screening programmes.

- Lesbian women have many known factors for smear abnormalities, yet are frequently told they do not need a cervical smear.
- Women's health services have been organized around contraception, disease control and fertility: lesbians may require all these services, but they have other needs that are not catered for (Nelson 1997).
- A third of lesbians may have an alcohol problem (Illman 1997).
- A woman with unacknowledged or unrecognized lesbian feelings may present with sexual or relationship problems.

Nursing issues

All clearly set out in guidelines produced by the RCN (1994) as *The Nursing Care of Lesbians and Gay Men*.

Spend some time thinking about the following:

- awareness that there is discrimination and prejudice towards lesbian patients
- awareness of the concerns that lesbians have about hostility and negative reactions from health care professionals once their sexuality is known
- understanding the importance of addressing the particular mental and physical health care needs of lesbians, especially adolescents
- using reflective practice to ensure unbiased and non-marginalizing behaviour
- examining own attitude to lesbian colleagues
- understanding the importance of ensuring equal opportunities and challenging homophobic behaviour
- remembering it is important not to make premature judgements about a person's sexual preference or behaviour
- many questions asked make an assumption of heterosexuality
- in order to avoid colluding with prejudices, giving reassurance that the same questions are asked of everyone with the aim of providing the best care (Curtis et al 1995)
- there are many concerns about confidentiality.

Key points

Assumptions are made that lesbians are not in need of sexual health advice or have fertility concerns or want babies.

REFERENCES

Curtis H, Hoolaghan T, Jewitt C (eds) 1995 Sexual health promotion in general practice. Radcliffe Medical Press, Oxford

Fairburn C, Dickerson M, Greenwood J 1983 Sexual problems and their management. Churchill Livingstone, Edinburgh

Hawton K, Harrison S 1997 Sexual problems. In: McPherson A, Waller D (eds) Women's health, 4th edn. Oxford University Press, Oxford, Ch 19

Illman L 1997 Promoting a healthy lifestyle. In: Andrews G (ed) Women's sexual health. Baillière Tindall, London, Ch 2

Jewitt C 1995 Sexual history taking in general practice. The HIV Project, London

Levy L 1998 Popping the question – taking sexual histories. Women's Health: The Journal for the Health Professional 3 (2): 22–24

Matthews P 1998 Sexual history taking in primary care. In: Carter Y, Moss C, Weyman A (eds) RCGP Handbook of Sexual Health in Primary Care. Royal College of General Practitioners, London, Ch 2

Nelson S 1997 Women's sexuality. In: Andrews G (ed) Women's sexual health. Baillière Tindall, London, Ch 1

RCN 1994 The nursing care of lesbians and gay men: An RCN Statement. Issues in nursing and health 26. Royal College of Nursing, London

RAPE

Rape and indecent assault are very serious offences. Rape is sexual intercourse, vaginal or anal, without the person's consent.

The Criminal Justice and Public Order Act (1994) amended the Sexual Offences Act (1956), recognizing that men can be raped. The Sexual Offences (Amendment) Bill (1992) ensures that a husband can be charged with raping his wife.

Indecent assault can be the insertion of objects into the vagina or the penis into other orifices.

'Rape is not an act of sex but an act of violence with sex as the primary weapon' (Craig 1990). Rape and other sexual offences are seriously under-reported for a number of reasons. Perhaps fewer than 10% of these offences is reported (Moore 1998).

Nursing issues

Guidance from the Royal College of Nursing (RCN 1995) recognizes the devastating effect that rape has on women.

Spend some time thinking about the following:

- always supporting the woman, while preserving any evidence (such as not washing or showering herself, or washing, or disposing of clothing or bedding)
- maintaining confidentiality and privacy, enabling the woman to feel safe and secure
- having regard and respect for the woman's age, race, culture, religion and sexuality
- being non-judgemental, non-directive and non-blaming – it is not her fault that she is in that situation and she can decide, if she wants, to:
  - undergo any tests or examination
  - inform the police

Nursing issues (continued)

- documenting any evidence of violence (e.g. bruising or bleeding)
- being able to describe the procedure for collecting forensic evidence
- having a knowledge of local and national services and resources
- being able to give the woman information and support in accessing
  - emergency contraception
  - testing for sexually transmitted infections (STI)
  - testing for HIV
  - crisis counselling
  - support groups
- the woman's partner may need support and counselling
- being alert for child protection issues (either that it is a child that has been raped, or that there are children at home at risk from the rapist).

A woman who has been raped may present years after the event with gynaecological problems, depression or other symptoms similar to post-traumatic stress disorder.

Nurses may see recently raped women:

- in Accident and Emergency departments
- admitted to hospital following severe injury
- in genitourinary medicine (GUM) clinics
- in family planning clinics.

For many women it can take weeks, months and often years for them to tell anyone of their experience of rape or sexual assault. It is impossible to estimate the effect that these experiences can have on all aspects of women's lives.

The nurse's initial reaction to a woman who has been raped or sexually assaulted can greatly affect the woman's feelings of guilt and self-worth (Harmond 1992).

WHAT TO DO

If the assault has been recent the raped woman should not wash, change her clothes, eat or have a drink before she is examined. The nurse should:

- believe the woman
- expect extremes of behaviour
- listen
- offer comfort
- discuss counselling or other support systems
- contact the police at the woman's request

- treat medical needs
- ensure safety (is she returning to a safe environment?) (Cole 1997).

NB: Do not use the word 'rape', instead use a phrase such as 'has someone had sex with you when you didn't want to?' It is possible that some women will only consider that they have been raped if it is carried out by a stranger or if violence has been used.

Possible examinations and tests are:

- all clothing worn at time of assault is removed and retained
- swabs taken from vagina, anus and mouth (for the assailant's semen or saliva)
- physical examination, including inspection of genital area and anus (for signs of injury)
- parings taken from nails (she may have scratched her assailant)
- blood samples (to match any stains on clothing or person of assailant (Gould 1990).

Tests at a GUM clinic may include those for:

- syphilis
- gonorrhoea
- *Chlamydia*
- *Trichomonas*
- hepatitis B
- HIV
- genital warts
- herpes.

MYTHS ABOUT RAPE

Society can be cruel about those who have been raped, suggesting that in some way they are responsible for what has happened. For example:

- 'she asked for it'
- 'she didn't really mean "no"'
- 'violent sex is enjoyable for the woman'
- 'she could have resisted'.

It is also commonly believed that it is usually carried out by a stranger and that it usually happens out of doors.

REFERENCES

Cole T 1997 Reaching out to help. Practice Nurse, 17 January, 33, 34, 36.
Craig DG 1990 Medicolegal problems in rape in the United Kingdom. In: Csanka GW, Oates JK (eds) Sexually transmitted diseases – a textbook of genitourinary medicine. Baillière Tindall, London.
Gould D 1990 Violence against women: sexual crimes. In: Gould D, Nursing care of women. Prentice Hall, London.
Harmond K 1992 Helping women after rape. Nursing Standard 6 (26): 44.
Moore L 1998 The experience of rape. Nursing Standard 12 (48): 49–56
RCN 1995 Responding to rape and sexual assault: guidance for good nursing practice. Issues in nursing and health 6. Royal College of Nursing, London

RESOURCES

Rape Crisis Centre, PO Box 69, London WC1, UK. Tel: 020 7837 1600.
Women Against Rape, PO Box 287, London NW6 5QU, UK. Tel.: 020 7837 7509.

SEXUAL ABUSE

Sexual abuse may be defined as any non-consensual, unwelcome or inappropriate sexual activity of any kind. It is usually carried out by men on women, frequently by the woman's partner. It is estimated to be seriously under-reported and is often carried out with escalating intrusiveness.

The abused woman may be exposed to indecent acts, pornography, photography, fondling, touching, masturbation (Hickerton 1997).

Sexual abuse is an abuse of power, and is carried out in all cultures and social settings. Sexual abuse can cause physical trauma to the genital tract, through violent penile penetration of vagina or anus.

Penetrating injuries, possibly with sharp objects, to the vagina can involve the bladder, rectum or peritoneal cavity and may be life-threatening.

The possibility of sexual abuse, particularly in a child or adolescent, should always be considered in cases of trauma (Pickrell 1997).

A woman who has been sexually abused is more likely to be at greater risk of (Ussher 1996):

- sexual dysfunction
- depression

- anxiety
- self-injurious behaviour
- attempted suicide.

Sexual dysfunction can result from sexual abuse and is characterized by (Hawton & Harrison 1997):

- low sexual desire
- sexual phobias
- problems of arousal.

Survivors of child sex abuse have shown links with (Reason 1998):

- low self-esteem
- inability to trust others
- sexual promiscuity
- prostitution
- difficulties in sexual and personal relationships
- eating disorders
- psychiatric illness (particularly female survivors of incest).

The long-term effects of child sexual abuse can vary greatly and may be related to (Reason 1998):

- age at onset of abuse
- duration of abuse
- closeness of relationship between child and abuser (e.g. worse with father or stepfather)
- degree of violence or threat of violence
- age difference
- absence of protective parent figures
- degree of secrecy.

Disclosure may be made in the setting of a routine but intimate consultation focusing on:

- cervical smear test
- vaginal discharge
- dysmenorrhoea
- dyspareunia
- antenatal clinic.

Many factors contribute to sexual abuse of daughters by fathers or stepfathers (Hawton & Harrison 1997):

- personality disorder in father
- alcohol abuse in father

- marital problems
- collusion of the mother.

Some questions to ask if abuse is suspected (Hickerton 1997):

- Do you feel safe in your current relationship?
- Do you feel your partner controls your behaviour too much?
- Have you ever been sexually or physically abused recently or as a child?
- Can you tell me what happened?

Nursing issues

Spend some time thinking about the following:

- awareness of sexual abuse as an issue
- awareness of the importance of always demonstrating sensitivity
- understanding issues of confidentiality
- understanding that an abused woman may not reveal the abuse for a long time, maybe even decades
- understanding the importance of believing what is revealed and being non-judgemental
- awareness of possible signs of abuse
- awareness of child protection issues arising from what an adult woman may reveal about her domestic or other relationships
- knowledge of local procedures if child sexual abuse is suspected
- respecting the fact that some women may not want to accept any help
- knowledge of access to specialist help, e.g. psychiatrist, clinical psychologist or counsellor
- knowledge of local and national information and resources.

Key point

There may be fertility issues as a result of trauma and/or infection.

REFERENCES

Hawton K, Harrison S 1997 Sexual problems. In: McPherson A, Waller D (eds) Women's health, 4th edn. Oxford University Press, Oxford, Ch 19
Hickerton M 1997 Women with special needs and concerns. In: Andrews G (ed) Women's sexual health. Baillière Tindall, London, Ch 5
Pickrell D 1997 Gynecological emergencies. In: Luesley D (ed) Common conditions in gynaecology. Chapman & Hall, London, Ch 3

Reason L 1998 Abuse, power and sex. In: Harrison T (ed) Children and sexuality. Baillière Tindall, London, Ch 7

Ussher J 1996 Female sexuality and reproduction. In: Niven C, Walker A (eds) Reproductive potential and fertility control. Butterworth-Heinemann, Oxford, Ch 11.

SEXUAL ANXIETIES AND DIFFICULTIES

Sexual anxieties and difficulties can lead to sexual dysfunction. **Sexual dysfunction** may be defined as the failure or impairment of sexual interest or response. There are different types of sexual dysfunction based on the three phases of the sexual response: sexual interest; arousal; orgasm. Primary sexual dysfunction is a problem that has been present from the onset of sexual activity. Secondary sexual dysfunction is a problem that occurs after a period of normal sexual function (Hawton & Harrison 1997).

Common presenting problems include:

- low sex drive (lack of sexual interest in self or partner)
- impaired arousal
- orgasmic dysfunction
- vaginismus (involuntary spasm of the pelvic floor muscles in anticipation of penetration and strong enough to prevent penetration)
- dyspareunia (pain with sexual intercourse)
- sexual fantasies and phobias.

HOW COMMON IS THE PROBLEM?

Thirty-three to 36% of women may have a sexual problem. It is estimated as many as 5% of all couples will not consummate a relationship within two years of marrying or living together (Parsons 1997).

Dyspareunia is painful penetrative sexual intercourse and can be due to (Skrine 1997):

- serious pelvic pathology
- an attack of thrush
- vaginal dryness from poor sexual technique
- emotional blocks to arousal.

CONTRIBUTING FACTORS

Several factors may contribute to sexual difficulties (Chamberlain 1995), including:

- dysfunctional family
- restrictive upbringing
- lack of sexual information
- incest/rape/traumatic sexual experience
- uncertain sexual identity
- ageing
- physical factors
- pregnancy/childbirth/parenthood
- response to life stresses
- guilt/poor self-image/body-image
- psychiatric disorders
- substance abuse (alcohol or drugs).

Other contributing causes can include (Christopher 1987):

- ignorance
- fear
- anxiety
- embarrassment, shame and disgust
- failure to communicate and unrealistic expectations
- collusive patterns in relationships.

Common medical problems in women may lead to sexual difficulties (Parsons 1997, Wakley, 1998). These include:

- arthritis – a pain-free position may be difficult to find
- cardiovascular disease – fear that it may bring on angina or another MI
- cancer of the cervix – after treatment there can be fear, guilt and shame
- colostomy or ileostomy – can affect body image and can produce feelings of disgust
- contraception – fear of pregnancy, shame and guilt at having sex
- chronic pelvic pain
- hysterectomy – fear on the part of the woman and her partner about damage during intercourse, may affect sex drive
- mental and physical disability – may not be considered as having sexual needs, may have limited opportunities

- mental illness, including depression – loss of sex drive is common, prescribed drugs may affect sexual functioning
- menopause – possible relationship problems, vaginal dryness is a common problem
- genital prolapse – sexual intercourse may be difficult and cause pain
- pelvic inflammatory disease and sexually transmitted infections – fear of pain may inhibit the sexual response, there may be guilt, shame and anger
- endometriosis – pain with sexual intercourse is a common problem
- any gynaecological cancer can affect body image and sexuality.

PRESENTATION

Sexual difficulties may be discovered as part of an on-going illness, or as a side-effect of treatment. They may be presented openly or as part of a 'while I'm here' for a related or unrelated problem, for example:

- contraceptive problems
- cervical smear
- infertility problems
- gynaecological problems, especially vaginal discharge
- following childbirth
- relationship, marital and family problems
- ambivalence about fertility.

They may be hidden by a psychosomatic complaint, such as headaches, backache or vaginal discharge (Christopher 1987, Wakley 1998).

There are nurses who are trained to carry out psychosexual counselling.

INFORMATION NEEDED AT FIRST ASSESSMENT (Hawton & Harrison 1997)

- The precise nature of the problem.
- The effect of the problem on the woman and her partner.
- Whether there is a major problem in the couple's general relationship.

- Whether she has had a satisfactory sexual relationship in the past.
- If she is adequately informed about sex.
- If there is any medical or psychiatric condition that might contribute to or cause the problem.
- If she is on any medication and what her alcohol consumption is.
- What changes she would like to achieve in her sexual adjustment.

Nursing issues

Spend some time thinking about the following:

- recognition that sexual problems may be accompanied by reticence and embarrassment on the part of both the health professional and the woman
- understanding of the importance of demonstrating sensitivity and respect
- knowledge of sexual functioning and emotional development
- awareness of own biases and prejudices
- awareness that treatment is by examining both the psychological and the physical aspects of the woman
- awareness of the importance of observing and using non-verbal communication
- knowledge of referral and access to local services, resources information, etc.

TREATMENT (Hawton & Harrison 1997)

- Counselling:
  - information, e.g. sexual anatomy, sexual response, affect of hysterectomy
  - advice, e.g. suitable positions for sex during pregnancy or recovering from a physical illness
  - permission-giving, e.g. normalizing some aspect of sexual behaviour about which there may be needless guilt, often masturbation or sexual fantasy.
- Sex therapy:
  - provided by those trained in psychosexual therapy
  - combines homework assignments, counselling and education
  - particularly effective for vaginismus and orgasmic dysfunction.

Where to refer

Referral facilities are shown in Box 7.1.

Box 7.1   Referral facilities for sexual problems (Wakley 1998)

Diagnosis	Referral facility
Part of a marital problem	Relate (formerly Marriage Guidance)
Part of a psychiatric illness	Psychiatrist
Long-standing personality problems or damage, e.g. survivor of childhood sexual abuse	Social worker/self-help group/psychologist
Focused psychosexual problem with an otherwise stable personality	Psychosexual clinic
Part of a general inability to cope with relationships	Counsellor/psychologist

---

Key points

- Use non-verbal communication, reflecting back feelings from the woman (i.e. 'you seem really uncomfortable, is there something I can help you with?') to open up the possibility of a sexual difficulty.
- Use open questions (i.e. 'you tell me that this difficulty started about six months age, can you tell me what else was going on in your life at that time?').
- Ensure mutual understanding, both of language and the nature of the problem.
- Remember that the woman knows how far she wants to go to resolve her sexual problems in a way that will best suit her and her partner (some people are not ready to confront difficulties).
- Men have sexual difficulties too.
- The problem can be very different from the initial complaint.
- Assessment of a sexual problem can have an important therapeutic function in itself.

REFERENCES

Chamberlain G (ed) 1995 Gynaecology by ten teachers, 16th edn. Arnold, London, Ch 11

Christopher E 1987 Sexuality & birth control in community work, 2nd edn. Tavistock, London

Hawton K, Harrison S 1997 Sexual problems. In: McPherson A, Waller D (eds) Women's health, 4th edn. Oxford University Press, Oxford, Ch 19

Parsons T 1997 Problems with sexuality. In: Luesley D (ed) Common conditions in gynaecology. Chapman & Hall Medical, London, Ch 14

Skrine R 1997 Blocks and freedoms in sexual life: a handbook of psychosexual medicine. Radcliffe Medical Press, Oxford

Wakley G 1998 Sexual problems in primary care. In: Carter Y, Moss C, Weyman A (eds) PCGP Handbook of Sexual Health in Primary Care. Royal College of General Practitioners, London, Ch 10

FURTHER READING

Hawton K, Harrison S 1997 Sexual problems. In: McPherson A, Waller D (eds) Women's health, 4th edn. Oxford University Press, Oxford

Penman J 1998 Action research in the care of patients with sexual anxieties. Nursing Standard 13 (13–15): 47–50

Skrine R 1997 Blocks and freedoms in sexual life: a handbook of psychosexual medicine. Radcliffe Medical Press, Oxford

Ussher JM 1996 Female sexuality and reproduction. In: Niven CA, Walker A (eds) Reproductive potential and fertility control. Butterworth-Heinemann, Oxford, Ch 11

Van Ooijen E, Charnock A 1994 Sexuality and patient care: a guide for nurses and teachers. Chapman & Hall, London

SEXUALITY

Sexuality is a woman's expression of herself as a sexual being; it is integral to her being. Whether or not she is sexually active is not an issue. It applies whatever her sexual orientation and whatever her state of health (Van Ooijen 1995).

HOW IS INDIVIDUAL SEXUALITY INFLUENCED?

Biological sex refers to male and female physical characteristics, while gender refers to how one is expected to behave as a woman or man, having different meanings in different cultures and times. Times of major social and biological change are vulnerable points (Nelson 1997), such as:

- puberty
- marriage
- pregnancy
- menopause.

CULTURE AND SEXUALITY (Pollen 1993)

- Assigning stereotypes is likely to offend.
- Even if very knowledgeable about the customs of ethnic minorities, never assume that all in this group adhere strictly to their cultural mores.

- Individuals have their own customs and rules.

SOCIETY AND SEXUALITY

Society can be ambivalent about or hostile to:

- adolescent sexuality
- teenage pregnancy
- premarital sex
- contraception
- abortion
- intentional childlessness
- large families in immigrant communities
- needs of those with learning difficulties
- diverse expressions of sexuality, e.g. lesbianism
- elderly people who are enjoying sex
- disabled people who are enjoying sex
- those who are ill or who live with chronic mental or physical conditions.

Nursing issues

Spend some time thinking about the following:

- understanding that no woman is asexual
- understanding that acknowledgment of an individual's sexuality is always relevant and an essential part of holistic care
- awareness of the impact of changed health status on body-image, self-esteem and the ability to participate in and enjoy future sexual relationships (Rafferty 1995)
- awareness of the importance of acquiring the necessary skills and confidence to address difficult or sensitive topics
- understanding how each woman thinks of herself as a woman and a sexual being to be able to give good sexual health care (Nelson 1997)
- to help women to address sexuality issues effectively, one needs to be aware of one's own values, attitudes and prejudices (Rafferty 1995)
- sexual care may embrace a spectrum from appearance and grooming to sexual dysfunction, most women's needs falling somewhere between the two (Rafferty 1995)
- thinking about the woman who says that she 'doesn't feel like a woman anymore' following her hysterectomy
- understanding that sexuality is not fixed throughout an individual's life, but changes during pregnancy, following childbirth and with ageing (Parsons 1997).

Think about the impact on a woman's sexuality of some other circumstances: the survivor of sexual abuse or the woman who has her sexual preference considered abnormal or deviant (e.g. lesbianism); the infertile woman who is not considered, by society, to be fulfilling her childbearing role; following surgery such as

- mastectomy
- hysterectomy
- formation of stoma
- amputation
- surgery for gynecological cancers
- any surgery that results in scarring
- for genital prolapse
- for urinary incontinence

– or following treatment for a sexually transmitted infection or following treatment for an abnormal smear, when a woman often feels dirty and guilty.

Living with a chronic debilitating disease (e.g. multiple sclerosis) affects sexuality, as does living with gross obesity or anorexia nervosa.

Key points

- There are social, cultural and political expectations and constraints about sexuality.
- Sexuality is bound up with secrecy, privacy, personal and moral codes.
- Sexuality is part of an individual's sense of identity and concept of self.
- Ignoring the sexual aspects of a woman's personality denies her holistic care.
- 'Patients' tend to be treated as asexual.

(Rafferty 1995)

Cancer itself does not cause sexual difficulties, but the concomitant physical, psychological and social factors may result in symptomatology (Ussher 1996).

GUIDELINES

Guidance for nurses on 'next-of-kin' for lesbian and gay patients and children with lesbian or gay parents (RCN 1998).

REFERENCES

Nelson S 1997 Women's sexuality. In: Andrews G (ed) Women's sexual health. Baillière Tindall, London, Ch 1

Parsons T 1997 Problems with sexuality. In: Luesley D (ed) Common conditions in gynaecology. Chapman & Hall, London, Ch 14

Pollen R 1993 Cultural perceptions and misconceptions. In: Montford H, Skrine R (eds) Contraceptive care. Chapman & Hall, London, Ch 9

Rafferty D 1995 Putting sexuality on the agenda. Nursing Times 91: 28–31

Royal College of Nursing 1998 Guidance for nurses on 'next-of-kin' for lesbian and gay patients and children with lesbian and gay parents. Issues in nursing and health 47. London.

Ussher J 1996 Female sexuality and reproduction. In: Niven C, Walker A (eds) Reproductive potential and fertility control. Butterworth-Heinemann, Oxford, Ch 11

Van Ooijen E 1995 How illness may affect patients' sexuality. Nursing Times 91: 36

FURTHER READING

Ashton G 1997 Sexuality during and after pregnancy. In: Andrews G (ed) Women's sexual health. Baillière Tindall, London, Ch 6

Nelson S 1997 Women's sexuality. In: Andrews G (ed) Women's sexual health. Baillière Tindall, London, Ch 1

Van Ooijen E, Charnock A 1994 Sexuality and patient care: a guide for nurses and teachers. Chapman & Hall, London

Wilton T 1998 Gender, sexuality and healthcare: improving services. In: Doyal L (ed) Women and health services. Open University Press, Buckingham, Ch 10

8

Common conditions and disorders

AMENORRHOEA

Amenorrhoea is the absence of any menstrual bleeding. 'To menstruate women require a functioning hypothalamic–pituitary–ovarian axis with a responding endometrium and genital outflow tract in the absence of endocrine or systemic disease or drug therapy, and in the presence of a normal chromosome complement' (Rees 1997). The causes of amenorrhoea are usually hormonal. There are two types:

- **Primary amenorrhoea**: a woman of any age who has never menstruated.
- **Secondary amenorrhoea**: the cessation of periods after menstruation has been established.

Amenorrhoea occurs in 10–20% of women complaining of infertility and is one of the commonest causes of referral to a gynaecological endocrine clinic (Franks 1987).

Physiological causes of amenorrhoea include:

- prepuberty
- pregnancy
- lactation
- post-menopause.

Fetal abnormalities in the development of ovaries, genital tract or external genitalia cause 60% of cases of primary amenorrhoea (Franks 1987). Forty per cent of women with secondary amenorrhoea have no developmental abnormality.

The most common causes of amenorrhoea are:

- Weight-related:
  - anorexia nervosa accounts for 15–33% of patients with amenorrhoea (Lockwood 1997)
  - body fat content seems to be significant as does a BMI below 19 (Rees 1997)

Table 8.1 Diagnosis in 100 consecutive women with secondary amenorrhoea seen in a gynaecological endocrine clinic (Franks 1987)

Diagnosis	No. of patients
Amenorrhoea related to weight loss	35
Polycystic ovary syndrome	32
Hyperprolactinaemia	11
Primary ovarian failure	11
Hypogonadotrophic hypogonadism (not weight-related)	9
Asherman's syndrome (uterine adhesions)	2

- also with intensive physical training in athletes and dancers (Drury 1994).
- Polycystic ovary syndrome (see p. 318).
- Hyperprolactinaemia (prolactin stimulates milk secretion; raised levels may indicate a hypothalamic pituitary disorder).

Other causes of amenorrhoea include:

- Hypothalamic–pituitary disorders (see Fig. 4.1):
  - pituitary tumour
  - hyperprolactinaemia
  - premature ovarian failure (premature menopause)
  - anorexia nervosa
  - prolonged periods of vigorous exercise (e.g. athletes, ballet dancers)
  - stress.
- Defects of ovary, uterus and vagina:
  - premature ovarian failure (menopause)
  - polycystic ovary syndrome (PCOS)
  - absence of uterus or vagina
  - imperforate hymen
  - gonadal dysgenesis (e.g. Turner's syndrome) (see p. 105).
- Other diseases:
  - thyroid disorder
  - adrenal disorder
  - severe or poorly controlled diabetes.
- Following radiotherapy or chemotherapy.
- Following hysterectomy.
- Chronic ill health (e.g. renal disease).
- Following childbirth, while breastfeeding.

Amenorrhoea may be encountered in:

- child development clinic
- school
- family planning clinic
- gynaecology clinic
- primary care.

Low levels of oestrogen increase the risk of osteoporosis. High levels of oestrogen (unopposed by progesterone as in PCOS) increase the risk of endometrial cancer.

Nursing issues

Spend some time thinking about the following:

- knowledge of the different types of amenorrhoea
- awareness of those who might be at risk
- understanding that it is always necessary to determine the cause of amenorrhoea
- awareness of the possible long-term consequences of som disorders causing amenorrhoea (e.g. osteoporosis, endometrial cancer)
- awareness of the anxiety and need for reassurance of the woman (and her family)
- considering issues around fertility and contraception (spontaneous or erratic ovulation is possible)
- encouraging a healthy lifestyle (e.g. in cases of eating disorder, over-exercising)
- ensuring access to information, resources, expert advice.

TREATMENT AND MANAGEMENT

Treatment is by trying to correct the underlying cause, when that has been identified.

Full history

The full history should be taken:

- age of menarche
- menstrual history prior to amenorrhoea
- development of secondary sex characteristics
- galactorrhoea (inappropriate milk-secretion from breasts)
- changes in weight or eating habits (possible eating disorder)
- medication (e.g. metaclopramide, phenothiazine, reserpine, methyldopa, cimetidine)
- family history of genetic abnormalities
- recent change in social or emotional circumstances, or psychological disturbance
- vigorous exercise
- hirsutism
- hot flushes, sweats, dry vagina
- previous pelvic surgery
- symptoms of endocrine disorder.

Assessment

Primary amenorrhoea

Any young woman not menstruating by 17 years should be investigated, or earlier if there has been no development of secondary sex characteristics. The physical examination of:

- stature (if short possibly Turner's syndrome)
- breasts (development means there has been some oestrogenic activity and the problem could be in the lower genital tract, if no development there could possibly be gonadal dysgenesis)
- external genitalia (for signs of pseudohermaphrodism)
- pelvis (imperforate hymen, short or absent vagina)
- hair distribution.

Investigations

Box 8.1 Investigations for amenorrhoea

Blood test	Possible outcome
Follicle-stimulating hormone (FSH)	Raised in primary ovarian failure
Serum prolactin	Hyperprolactinaemia due to prolactinoma (temporary increase can be due to stress)
Oestrogen	Deficiency in hypogonadotrophic hypogonadism
Luteinizing hormone (LH)	Raised in polycystic ovarary syndrome (with raised serum testosterone and reversed FSH/LH ratio)
Chromosomal studies	Turner's syndrome or mosaicism
Testosterone	High with testicular feminization

Other investigations

- Progestogen challenge (vaginal bleeding after a short course of progestogen) – a positive result will demonstrate:
  - sufficient oestrogen production to stimulate the endometrium
  - a responsive endometrium
  - a patent vagina.
- Pelvic ultrasound can demonstrate:
  - presence, size and appeearence of uterus

- size of ovaries, and presence and size of follicles.
- Urogram, when there are uterine or vaginal malformations – associated abnormalities of ureters and kidneys.
- Skull X-ray or CT scan, when prolactin raised to exclude pituitary tumour.
- Laparoscopy and ovarian biopsy to identify primordial oocytes.

Treatment

Treatment will depend on what caused the amenorrhoea and whether the woman wants to be pregnant. If amenorrhoea is judged to be caused by stress or an emotional problem, spontaneous recovery is to be expected if the problem can be removed or alleviated by the passage of time (Chamberlain 1995).

Primary amenorrhoea

If the uterus is present hormones are used to induce menstruation.

Secondary amenorrhoea

Ability to induce menstruation will depend on:

- the state of the endometrium
- the hypothalamic–pituitary–ovarian axis (this can be influenced by drug therapy).

FERTILITY

Conception can only occur if there is ovarian tissue with primary ovarian follicles. Menstruation, ovulation and fertility can be restored in patients using drugs (Rees 1997).

Surgical treatments could include

- removal of hymen
- reconstruction of vagina
- removal of testes in testicular feminization – if left there is a 50% chance of malignancy (Rees 1997).

Key points

Oestrogen is essential for:

- development of secondary sexual characteristics
- skeletal development.

The effects of stress on the menstrual cycle should never be underestimated.

In both primary and secondary amenorrhoea:

- pregnancy must be excluded
- underweight is significant.

REFERENCES

Chamberlain G 1995 (ed) Gynaecology by ten teachers, 16th edn. Arnold, London, Ch 8

Drury PL 1994 Endocrinology. In: Kumar P, Clark M (eds) Clinical medicine, 3rd edn. Saunders, London, Ch 16

Franks S 1987 Primary and secondary amenorrhoea. British Medical Journal 294: 815–819

Lockwood G 1997 Infertility and early pregnancy loss. In: McPherson A, Waller D (eds) Women's health, 4th edn. Oxford University Press, Oxford, Ch 8

Rees M 1997 Menstrual problems. In: McPherson A, Waller D (eds) Women's health, 4th edn. Oxford University Press, Oxford, Ch 10

FURTHER READING

Rees M 1997 Menstrual problems. In: McPherson A, Waller D (eds) Women's health, 4th edn. Oxford University Press, Oxford, Ch 10

Steele J 1997 Common gynaecological problems. In: Andrews G (ed) Women's sexual health. Baillière Tindall, London, Ch 16

BENIGN BREAST DISORDERS

Benign breast disorders usually include one of the following:

- lumps (commonly fibroadenoma or cysts)
- pain
- nipple discharge.

WHY ARE THEY A PROBLEM?

Benign breast disorders are very common, but they must be differentiated from the much less common breast cancers.

- Breast cancer is the commonest malignant condition to affect women (see p. 251).
- Breast diseases of all sorts account for a substantial number of consultations each year in general practice.
- Each year a general practitioner (GP) can expect to see around 30 new presentations per 1000 women relating to breast disease.
- Only 5.8% of women presenting to their GP with a breast disorder are found to have breast cancer (Austoker et al 1997).

Nursing issues

Spend some time thinking about the following:

- knowledge of common breast disorders
- knowledge of breast awareness and how to communicate it (see p. 30)
- knowledge of the National Breast Screening Programme (see p. 32)
- knowledge of referral criteria
- awareness of the anxiety and fear that many women will experience before a differential diagnosis has been made
- awareness of the extreme effects of severe breast pain on some women's lives and relationships
- understanding issues of accountability: e.g. carrying out breast examination only after undertaking specialist training (RCN 1995)
- knowledge to provide information and support for women, e.g. self-help advice
- it is not the nurse's role to provide a diagnosis or to imply that she or he can in any way define whether a woman may or may not have breast cancer (RCN 1995)
- any woman presenting with breast pain should have a history taken and be examined to exclude any discrete mass.

WHEN TO REFER

The National Health Service Breast Screening Programme (NHSBSP) has produced guidelines for general practitioners for the referral of patients with breast problems to a specialist (Austoker et al 1995). Conditions that require referral are:

- Lump:
  - any new discrete lump
  - new lump in pre-existing nodularity
  - asymmetrical nodularity that persists at review after menstruation
  - abscess
  - cyst persistently refilling or recurrent cyst.

- Pain:
  - if associated with a lump
  - intractable pain not responding to reassurance, simple measures such as wearing a well supporting bra, and common drugs (e.g. gamolenic acid)
  - unilateral breast pain in post-menopausal women.
- Nipple discharge:
  - all women aged 50 and over
  - women under 50 with:
    bilateral discharge sufficient to stain clothes
    blood stained discharge
    persistent single duct discharge.
- Nipple retraction or distortion, nipple eczema.
- Change in skin contour.
- Family history: when requested by a woman with a strong family history of breast cancer.

Women who can be managed, at least initially, by their general practitioner (Austoker et al 1995) are:

- young women with tender, lumpy breasts and older women with symmetrical nodularity, provided that they have no localized abnormality
- women with minor and moderate degrees of breast pain who do not have a discrete palpable lesion
- women aged under 50 who have nipple discharge that is from more than one duct or is intermittent and is neither bloodstained nor troublesome.

NODULARITY

Nodularity is (Dixon & Mansel 1995):

- an area of lumpiness
- ill-defined
- often bilateral
- tends to fluctuate with the menstrual cycle.

BREAST LUMPS

Breast lumps can be (Austoker et al 1995):

- Fibroadenomas:

- account for 12% of all palpable, symptomatic breast lumps
- very common in 15–30 age group
- spherical, rubbery, smooth and very mobile ('breast mouse')
- 5% will grow progressively, 20% will regress, the majority will stay the same size
- diagnosis is by clinical examination, ultrasound and fine needle aspiration cytology
- can be safely left in situ after the diagnosis has been made, though some women request surgical excision.
- Cysts:
  - most common in 40–50 years age group
  - in 50% of women they are multiple
  - most often in upper outer quadrant
  - commonest abnormality in patients presenting at a breast clinic
  - frequently asymptomatic, but may be painful
  - diagnosis and management is by aspiration (with or without ultrasound) and re-examination to ensure no residual mass exists
  - 10% of cysts refill to become palpable
  - 50% of women with a cyst will develop another cyst elsewhere in the breast.

BREAST PAIN (MASTALGIA)

- Most mastalgia is of minor or moderate severity and is accepted as part of the normal changes that occur in relation to the menstrual cycle (Mansel 1995).
- Mastalgia is cyclical (before menstruation) or non-cyclical.
- Completion of a breast pain record chart will differentiate between the two.

Cyclical mastalgia

Cyclical mastalgia:

- is the commonest mastalgia (75%)
- occurs at average age 35
- is relieved by the menopause
- may continue, off and on, for years

- is often associated with areas of nodularity
- its course is not affected by pregnancy, oral contraceptives and parity
- physical activity can increase the pain.

Non-cyclical mastalgia

Non-cyclical mastalgia:

- is seen in older women
- is not related to the menstrual cycle
- the pain may arise from the breast or be musculoskeletal in origin
- there may be localized chest wall pain or a localized single tender area (trigger spot)
- may respond to non-steroidal anti-inflammatory drugs (NSAIDs) and wearing a firm, supporting bra for 24 hours a day
- a localized tender area may respond to an injection of local anaesthetic and steroid.

Treatment and management of cyclical mastalgia

Mild to moderate mastalgia:

- examination and reassurance
- 85% respond to reassurance that they do not have cancer
- self-help remedies may be effective (Box 8.2).

Gamolenic acid (contained in evening primrose oil and starflower oil):

- is an essential fatty acid

Box 8.2 Analgesia

- changing or refitting bra (many women wear incorrectly fitting bras)
- reduction of intake of caffeine and saturated fats (although the role of these in breast pain is unclear)
- gamolenic acid (in evening primrose oil) can give a good response
- stopping oral contraceptive or hormone replacement may help, but may present other problems

---

- women with mastalgia are found to have abnormal plasma fatty acid profiles
- reduces pain, tenderness and nodularity in 60% of women at a dose of 300 mg daily (Austoker et al 1997)
- there may be a slow response, so treatment should be continued for at least 4 months
- has minimal side-effects
- has no effect on the menstrual cycle
- can be used with oral contraception
- if there is a good response treatment is for <6 months, if breast pain recurs (in half of those who responded) it is usually milder, otherwise treatment can be repeated.

Moderate to severe mastalgia

Moderate to severe mastalgia may affect the quality of life of 15% of women with mastalgia, e.g. sleep, daily activities, employment, sexual and social relationships, sport and exercise. NHSBSP protocol (Austoker et al 1995) for treating moderate to severe mastalgia is as follows:

- gamolenic acid is the first-line treatment
- if there is no response:
  - danazol (inhibits pituitary gonadotrophins) (Box 8.3)
  - bromocriptine (inhibits release of prolactin by the pituitary) (Box 8.3)
  - both drugs should be used with non-hormonal contraception
  - if there is not a response to one of the drugs, it does not mean that there will not be a response to the other
  - it is always necessary to assess the severity of the symptoms before starting hormonal treatment and for full counselling to be given about expected side-effects

---

Box 8.3   Danazol and bromocriptine in the treatment of mastalagia

Danazol	*Bromocriptine*
• Can relieve symptoms in 70% of women • Side-effects include nausea, hirsutism, acne and weight gain	• >20% of women treated will have side-effects sufficient to stop treatment, e.g. nausea, vomiting, constipation, dizziness

---

Key points

- Benign breast problems can usually be managed in primary care.
- Referral to a specialist is essential if it is not possible to differentiate the diagnosis.
- There are ineffective treatments for breast pain and there is no evidence that some commonly used treatments work:
  - diuretics
  - pyridoxine (vitamin B_6)
  - antibiotics
  - progestogens.
- Breast pain of any type is a rare symptom of breast cancer.
- Only 7% of patients with breast cancer have mastalgia as their only symptom (Mansel 1995).

- other drugs (e.g. tamoxifen and a gonadotrophin-releasing hormone agonist) have been used to some effect, but would only be available from a specialist clinic.

REFERENCES

Austoker J, Mansel R, Baum M et al 1995 Guidelines for referral of patients with breast problems. NHSBSP, Sheffield

Austoker J, McPherson A, Clarke J, Lucassen A 1997 Breast problems. In: McPherson A, Waller D (eds) Women's health, 4th edn. Oxford University Press, Oxford, Ch 5

Dixon JM, Mansel RE 1995 Symptoms, assessment, and guidelines for referral. In: Dixon JM (ed) ABC of breast diseases. BMJ Publishing, London

Mansel RE 1995 Breast pain. In: Dixon JM (ed) ABC of breast diseases. BMJ Publishing, London

RCN 1995 Breast palpation and breast awareness: guidelines for practice. Issues in nursing and health 35. Royal College of Nursing, London

---

FURTHER READING

Dixon JM (ed) 1995 ABC of breast diseases. BMJ Publishing, London
Stoppard M 1998 Breast health. Dorling Kindersley, London

RESOURCES

Breast Care Campaign (leaflets), Blythe Hall, Blythe Road, London W14 0HB, UK.

BREAST CANCER

In the UK:

- It is the commonest cancer in minority ethnic groups.
- It is the commonest cause of cancer mortality in women (18%).
- 1 in 12 women will develop breast cancer at some time in their lives.
- 80% of cases occur in post-menopausal women, but there are still 7000 cases each year in pre-menopausal women.
- Each year more than 1000 women are diagnosed with breast cancer while pregnant, lactating or during the first post-partum year.
- It is the commonest single cause of all deaths in women aged 35–54 years.
- Breast cancer deaths account for 20% of all female cancer deaths.
- In 1995 14 080 women died from breast cancer (Cancer Research Campaign 1996).
- In 1993 of 110 000 women diagnosed with cancer, breast cancer accounted for 28% of all cancers in women (ONS 1999).

CAUSES

The causes of breast cancer are not known. Breast screening aims to increase earlier diagnosis and reduce mortality (see p. 32). Some risk factors are recognized as having an association with breast cancer.

Risk factors

Risk factors with an established association:

- age (more likely in the older woman, over the age of 50)
- early menarche (onset of menstruation before age 11)
- late menopause (after age 54)
- nulliparity (no children)
- first child after the age of 30
- family history (see p. 253)
- previous benign breast disease (atypical hyperplasia)

- cancer in the other breast
- exposure to ionizing radiation.

Hormonal factors

Combined oral contraceptive:

- Small increased risk in those currently taking or who have recently stopped the pill.
- Increased risk disappears 10 years after stopping (Collaborative Group 1996).
- Minimal risk for short-term use before first pregnancy and long-term use in those who have had children.
- Risk of long-term use (more than 5 years) before first full-term pregnancy is not known (Austoker et al 1997).
- Theory is that the oral contraceptives stimulate an existing tumour, rather than initiating the cancer (Austoker et al 1997).
- The benefits of this reliable method of contraception need to be considered.

Hormone replacement therapy (HRT):

- There is a small increased risk with longer-term use (5–15 years).
- The association is not well understood.
- Cancers that develop while a woman is taking HRT tend to be found at an earlier stage and be more amenable to treatment (Collaborative Group 1997).
- The long-term benefits of HRT, particularly in relation to bone fracture risk and cardiovascular disease, need to be considered.
- Breast density can increase with HRT, which can make detection of breast cancers more difficult (McPherson et al 1995).

Other possible risk factors

- Socio-economic status (incidence is higher in social class 1 and 2).
- Lifestyle:
  - diet high in saturated fat, perhaps during early life (although the evidence is inconclusive)

- obesity in post-menopausal women (whereas obesity in young women reduces the risk)
- high alcohol consumption (although the relationship is inconsistent) (McPherson et al 1995).

Protective factors

Some forms of behaviour may protect against breast cancer (Cancer Research Campaign 1996):

- high levels of physical activity
- breast feeding
- a diet high in fibre, fruit and vegetables.

FAMILY HISTORY

Up to 10% of breast cancer is due to genetic susceptibility (Cancer Research Campaign 1996):

- It is the susceptibility that is inherited, not cancer itself.
- It can be transmitted through either parent.
- It is possible for family members to transmit the gene without developing cancer themselves.
- BRCA1 and BRCA2 are the two breast cancer genes that so far have been identified.
- BRCA1 is associated with an increased risk of ovarian cancer.
- The risk increases when one first degree relative (mother, sister, daughter) has breast cancer, and increases considerably when two are affected.
- The risk increases if the relative has bilateral disease and if the disease occurs at a young age.
- Familial breast cancers can also be associated with ovary, colon and prostate cancer.

SYMPTOMS

- The commonest presentation is a lump, found by the woman or her partner.
- Anything that is different from a woman's normal cyclical changes:
  - change in shape or size of breast

- a new lump
- change in skin contour
- unusual pain
- nipple retraction or distortion, discharge or eczema.

DIAGNOSIS (see Box 8.4)

Usually by a combination of:

- mammography
- ultrasound
- fine needle aspiration
- core biopsy.

Box 8.4 Investigations carried out by specialist

Breast lump
Triple assessment:
- clinical examination
- imaging (mammography and/or ultrasound)
- fine needle aspiration cytology (+/– core biopsy).

Breast pain
Unilateral persistent mastalgia:
- mammography or ultrasonography.

Localized areas of painful nodularity:
- mammography or ultrasonography.

Focal lesions:
- fine needle aspiration cytology.

Nipple discharge
Clinical examination and mammography.

Nipple retraction
Clinical examination and mammography.

Change in skin contour
Clinical examination, mammography and ultrasound.
(Austoker et al 1995)

TREATMENT

The aim of the treatment is to remove local disease and to prevent recurrence, and limit the spread of metastases.

Most patients will have a combination of local treatments to control local disease and systemic treatment for any micrometastatic disease (Sainsbury et al 1995).

Treatment is usually managed by a combination of:

- surgery
- radiotherapy
- chemotherapy
- hormone therapy.

Treatment will largely depend on the staging of the disease and the woman's wishes.

Most breast cancers arise from the epithelial cells lining the milk ducts:

- Ductal carcinoma in situ (DCIS) – the cancer remains within the basement membrane and is considered non-invasive.
- Stage 1 – the tumour is less than 2 cm, and confined to the breast.
- Stage 2 – the tumour is 2–5 cm, axillary lymph nodes may be involved.
- Stage 3 – the tumour may be larger than 5 cm, the chest wall and regional nodes may be involved.
- Stage 4 – distant metastases are to be found, usually in lungs, liver and bones.

Other tests when breast cancer has been diagnosed:

- blood test for full blood count (FBC) and liver function
- chest X-ray
- if more advanced disease is suspected then ultrasound of liver and bone scan.

The outlook after diagnosis

Survival will depend on:

- stage of the disease
- grade of tumour (differentiation from normal breast tissue)
- presence of high concentrations of oestrogen receptors (ER+ve) indicating a tumour that requires oestrogen for continued growth and predicting a response to hormonal manipulation (Miller et al 1995)
- age at diagnosis (outcome poorer if aged under 35).

Survival also depends on the treatment and management given, and whether or not it was given in a specialist unit.

Survival at 5 years of patients according to stage of tumour:

- stage 1   84%
- stage 2   71%
- stage 3   48%
- stage 4   18%.

Survival at 10 years according to involvement of axillary lymph nodes (Miller et al 1995):

- all patients   45.9%
- negative nodes   64.9% (i.e. with no lymph node
  involvement)
- positive nodes   24.9% (with lymph node involvement)
- 1–3 nodes   37.5%
- >4 nodes   13.4%.

Nursing issues

Spend some time thinking about the following:

- awareness of the incidence of breast cancer
- understanding the importance of promoting breast awareness and the uptake of breast screening
- understanding the importance of the prompt detection, diagnosis and treatment of breast cancer
- awareness of the impact of breast cancer on a woman's body image, sexuality, family and other relationships
- awareness of issues around fertility, for those who have not started or completed their family
- treating with respect and sensitivity those who present with advanced disease, having denied symptoms out of fear or ignorance
- knowledge of treatment and management options, including length of treatment and expected and possible side-effects
- knowledge of local and national resources, including ensuring access to a specialist breast care nurse
- awareness of the variability in the quality of cancer treatments throughout the country.

Research

At many centres there is ongoing research:

- to improve the prevention and earlier detection of breast cancer
- to improve and develop new techniques in chemotherapy and hormone therapy.

> **Key points**
>
> - Non-symptomatic cancers detected at routine screening are smaller and more likely to be non-invasive (Blamey et al 1995).
> - The earlier that breast cancer is diagnosed and treated, the better the outcome.
> - Breast reconstruction following mastectomy:
>   - can sometimes be carried out at the time of the mastectomy
>   - may be carried out months or even years later.
> - Lymphoedema of the arm can be a problem following breast cancer. This is because the lymphatic system can be damaged by surgery to remove axillary lymph nodes, by radiotherapy or by disease recurrence. Also, after the removal of axillary lymph nodes the arm on the affected side is much more susceptible to infection; therefore, advice should be given about prevention (e.g. avoiding scratches, wearing gloves for household tasks) (CancerBACUP 1998).

GUIDELINES

Improving Outcomes in Breast Cancer produced by the Cancer Guidance Sub-Group of the Clinical Outcomes Group (The Department of Health, Literature Line 0800 555 777). *The Management of Primary Breast Cancer*:

- Survival rates for women with breast cancer in England and Wales are worse than in most European countries (the guidance notes do not mention Northern Ireland or Scotland).
- There are wide variations in the management of breast cancer within the country.
- The speed and cost-effectiveness of accurate diagnosis of breast cancer can be increased by using a combination of clinical examination, mammography and fine needle aspiration cytology (triple assessment).
- The use of triple assessment will reduce the number of women needing surgical biopsy.
- Women are less anxious when they are given full verbal and written information about their treatment, and opportunities to discuss options with clinical staff.
- It is recognized that doctors may overestimate the amount of information that they communicate and that is understood by the woman
- Research suggests that psychosocial interventions can improve quality and length of life.
- Mastectomy and breast-conserving surgery plus radiotherapy have similar survival rates.
- Breast-conserving surgery leads to better preservation of body image but local recurrence rates are higher.
- The use of adjuvant systemic therapy with tamoxifen, ovarian ablation, or chemotherapy improves survival and recurrence rates in most groups of women and is highly cost-effective.

- There is no evidence that routine intensive hospital follow-up, apart from regular mammography, improves outcomes after primary treatment compared with GP-led follow-up with ready access to specialist care when needed.
- The management of breast cancer, and its outcomes, can be improved if care is provided by specialists working in multi-disciplinary teams with a sufficient number of new cases each year (Effective Health Care 1996).

REFERENCES

Austoker J, Mansel R, Baum M et al 1995 Guidelines for referral of patients with breast problems. NHS Breast Screening Programme, Sheffield

Austoker J, McPherson A, Clarke J, Lucassen A 1997 Breast problems. In: McPherson A, Waller D (eds) Women's health, 4th edn. Oxford University Press, Oxford, Ch 5

Blamey RW, Wilson ARM, Patnick J 1995 Screening for breast cancer. In: Dixon JM (ed) ABC of breast diseases. BMJ Publishing, London

CancerBACUP 1998 Understanding cancer of the breast. London

Cancer Research Campaign 1996 Breast cancer – UK. Factsheet 6

Collaborative Group on Hormonal Factors in Breast Cancer 1996 Breast cancer and hormonal contraceptives: collaborative reanalysis of individual data on 53 297 women with breast cancer and 100 239 women without breast cancer from 54 epidemiological studies. Lancet 347: 1713–1727

Collaborative Group on Hormonal Factors in Breast Cancer 1997 Breast cancer and hormone replacement therapy: collaborative reanalysis of data from 51 epidemiological studies of 52 705 women with breast cancer and 108 411 women without breast cancer. Lancet 350: 1047–1059

Effective Health Care 1996 The management of primary breast cancer. NHS Centre for Reviews and Dissemination, York

McPherson K, Steele CM, Dixon JM 1995 Breast cancer – epidemiology, risk factors, and genetics. In: Dixon JM (ed) ABC of breast diseases. BMJ Publishing, London

Miller WR, Ellis IO, Sainsbury JRC 1995 Prognostic factors. In: Dixon JM (ed) ABC of breast diseases. BMJ Publishing, London.

Office for National Statistics 1999 Cancer registration in England and Wales 1993. ONS, London

Sainsbury JRC, Anderson TJ, Morgan DAL 1995 Breast cancer. In: Dixon JM (ed) ABC of breast diseases. BMJ Publishing, London

FURTHER READING

Curling G, Tierney K 1997 Breast screening and breast disorders. In: Andrews G (ed) Women's sexual health. Baillière Tindall, London, Ch 10

Denton S 1996 Breast cancer nursing. Chapman & Hall, London

Dixon JM (ed) 1995 ABC of breast diseases. BMJ Publishing, London

Stoppard M 1998 Breast health. Dorling Kindersley, London

RESOURCES

CancerBACUP, 3 Bath Place, Rivington Street, London EC2A 3DR, UK.
Cancer Support Service, Tel.: 020 7613 2121. Freeline (for calls from outside
London) 0800 18 11 99.

CERVICAL CANCER

Cervical cancer is malignant change in the cells of the squamo-
columnar junction, where the squamous cells of the exocervix
meet the columnar cells of the endocervix (see Fig. 2.1). This is the
area referred to as the transformation zone (TZ) from which the
cervical smear is taken (see p. 35). Metaplasia is the normal
process by which the columnar cells are replaced by squamous
epithelium.

Cervical cancer can be prevented by early detection and
treatment of preinvasive disease (Luesley 1997). Invasive
carcinoma is preceded by premalignant lesions, known collec-
tively as cervical intraepithelial neoplasia (CIN): CIN 3 or severe
dysplasia is coded as carcinoma *in situ* (Cancer Research
Campaign 1994). The majority of cervical cancers are squamous
cell carcinomas.

Adenocarcinoma was rare but is now becoming more
common, especially among younger women where it may make
up more than 20% of cervical cancers (McPherson & Austoker
1997).

INCIDENCE

- In England in 1998–99 around 4000 new cases of invasive
  carcinoma of the cervix were registered (DOH 1999).
- It is the eighth commonest cancer in women.
- 15.5% of these cases were in women under 35 years, and it
  was the commonest cancer in this age group.
- A further 22 000 women were registered with carcinoma *in
  situ*.
- 85% of those with carcinoma *in situ* were aged under 45 years.
- There has been a substantial decrease in the mortality rate in
  the last 20 years, but little change in the incidence (Cancer
  Research Campaign 1994).

- Deaths from cervical cancer:
  - have fallen from >2000 in the 1970s to <1400 in 1994
  - 95% are in women aged over 35
  - the fall in death rate is due to a fall in the deaths from squamous cell carcinoma (McPherson and Austoker 1997).

CAUSES

Exact causes have not been identified, but some risk factors are known. These are:

- Young age at first sexual intercourse.
- Number of sexual partners (possibly because of a carcinogen in seminal fluid, however there is no reliable evidence to support this).
- Low socio-economic group.
- Smoking.
- History of a sexually transmitted infection – particularly human papilloma virus (HPV); HPV types 16 and 18 have a strong association.
- Method of contraception:
  - barrier method may protect
  - use of oral contraceptive for more than 5 years may increase risk (McPherson and Austoker 1997).
- Never having had a cervical smear – prior to 1988 two-thirds of those diagnosed with invasive carcinoma had never had a smear (Cancer Research Campaign 1994).

SYMPTOMS

There may be none in early disease, the abnormality being picked up on routine cervical screening. Noticeable symptoms include:

- irregular vaginal bleeding
- post-coital bleeding (bleeding after sexual intercourse)
- offensive discharge
- pain – this develops late and indicates extension of the growth beyond the limits of the cervix: lower abdominal pain or pain felt over the sacrum (Chamberlain 1995).

DIAGNOSIS

Diagnosis is:

- on a cervical smear
- by biopsy.

SURVIVAL

Survival depends on how far the invasive cancer has spread:

Stage I   is confined to the cervix
Stage II   has spread beyond the cervix but not onto the pelvic floor
Stage III   has spread onto the pelvic floor
Stage IV   has spread more widely (McPherson & Austoker 1997).

Overall survival rate for invasive carcinoma is 57%:

Stage I   79%
Stage II   47%
Stage III   22%
Stage IV   7%.
(Cancer Research Campaign 1994)

TREATMENT

Treatment will depend on the stage of the disease:

- In pre-cancerous conditions the abnormal cells can be destroyed by various methods:
  - cryotherapy (freezing)
  - cold coagulation (heat)
  - diathermy
  - laser therapy
  - cone biopsy (see p. 342).
- Localized early cancer:
  - surgery alone (probably a radical hysterectomy) (see p. 332)
  - surgery followed by radiotherapy, because of involvement of pelvic lymph nodes in 20% of women (Redman 1997).

- Advanced disease – radiotherapy and/or chemotherapy sometimes followed by surgery.

Nursing issues

Spend some time thinking about the following:

- knowledge of the workings of the National Cervical Screening Programme (see p. 35)
- understanding the importance of promoting a lifestyle that will reduce the risks from factors known to increase the risk of cervical cancer
- understanding the importance of promoting regular cervical smears as a means of intervening in the progression of the disease
- awareness of the feelings of those who perceive cervical cancer as 'dirty' and the result of 'bad' sexual behaviour
- awareness of the possible effects on a woman's sexuality and sexual relationships
- awareness of the guilt, fear and embarrassment that prevent some women from attending for a cervical smear or from reporting prolonged symptoms
- understanding the importance of the person taking the cervical smear being appropriately trained (RCN 1994).

CERVICAL INTRAEPITHELIAL NEOPLASIA

Cervical intraepithelial neoplasia (CIN) is the term used to describe preinvasive disease of the cervix. There are three grades to describe the disease, based on histological examination of a biopsy. The grading is made according to the proportion of epithelium occupied by abnormal cells (Box 8.5):

Box 8.5	Grading of CIN
CIN 1	• a third of the cells in the affected area are abnormal • generally at the low-risk end of the spectrum • may be treated or kept under close surveillance.
CIN 2	• up to two-thirds of the cells in the affected area are abnormal • at intermediate risk • should be treated once diagnosed.
CIN 3	• all the cells in the affected area are abnormal • at high risk of progression to invasive disease • should be treated once diagnosed.

Nursing issues

Spend some time thinking about the following:

- understanding and being able to explain all terminology
- being aware of the local method of management
- encouraging a healthy lifestyle (especially stopping smoking)
- supporting the woman through her treatment
- awareness of many women's perception that cervical disease is 'dirty' and the result of 'bad' sexual behaviour
- awareness of the possible effect on a woman's sexuality and sexual relationships
- awareness of the shame, fear and guilt that can prevent women attending for screening or reporting symptoms
- ensuring understanding of the importance of continuing surveillance and follow-up
- ensuring systems are in place to prevent 'losing' the woman.

Treatment (see p. 339)

Treatment aims to remove or destroy abnormal cells found in the transformation zone of the cervix.

- Extremes of heat or cold are equally effective.
- Some methods of treatment will require more than one visit.
- Cervical function is not affected by the destructive therapies and LLETZ.
- The woman may experience painful uterine contractions. This will depend on the type and extent of the treatment and may last for 1–2 days (aspirin, paracetamol or non-steroidal anti-inflammatory drugs (NSAIDs) should be adequate).
- Local anaesthetic is often used.
- Hysterectomy would rarely be used as treatment for CIN.

Key points

- It is not known what proportion will progress to pre-cancer and cancer, how long it may take and what may affect the progression.
- The grades in precancer are stages in a continuing process.
- Palliative treatment is as important as treatment intended to cure (Redman 1997)
- Not all pre-cancers will eventually progress to cancer if left untreated.
- CIN 1 can revert to normal.
- Some CIN will remain stationary and not progress.
- It is impossible to predict any one individual's outcome if untreated.

Local destructive therapy

- Carbon dioxide laser ablation
- 'cold' coagulation
- cryosurgery
- electrocoagulation.

Local excision

- Knife cone biopsy
- laser cone biopsy
- large loop excision of the transformation zone (LLETZ).

REFERENCES

Cancer Research Campaign 1994 Cancer of the cervix uteri. Factsheet 12
Chamberlain G (ed) 1995 Gynaecological tumours. In: Gynaecology by ten
   teachers, 16th edn. Arnold, London
Department of Health 1999 Cervical screening programme 1998–99. Bulletin
   1999/32. DOH, London
Luesley D 1997 The abnormal cervical smear. In: Luesly D (ed) Common
   conditions in gynaecology. Chapman & Hall, London, Ch 9
McPherson A, Austoker J 1997 Cervical cytology. In: McPherson A, Waller D
   (eds) Women's Health, 4th edn. Oxford University Press, Oxford, Ch 12
RCN 1994 Cervical screening: guidelines for good practice. Issues in nursing and
   health 28. Royal College of Nursing, London
Redman C 1997 Gynaecological cancers. In: Luesley D (ed) Common conditions
   in gynaecology. Chapman & Hall, London, Ch 10

FURTHER READING

Austoker J, Davey C 1997 Cervical smear results explained: a guide for primary
   care. Cancer Research Campaign, London
Cancer BACUP 1995 Understanding cancer of the cervix. London
Gould D 1990 Neoplasms of the female genital tract. In: Gould D, Nursing care
   of women. Prentice Hall, New York, Ch 12

RESOURCES

CancerBACUP, 3 Bath Place, Rivington Street, London EC2A 3JR, UK.
Cancer Information Service, Tel: 020 7613 2121. Freeline (for calls from outside
   London) 0800 18 11 99.

CHRONIC PELVIC PAIN

Chronic pelvic pain is defined as pain in the pelvic region, which
has persisted for more than 6 months and is not relieved by

non-narcotic analgesics (Wiener 1994). Other pathology has been excluded, by history and examination, and by investigation.

The pelvic pain has typical characteristics:

- a persistent dull ache made worse by posture (e.g. standing, walking)
- dysmenorrhoea
- dyspareunia (painful sexual intercourse)
- post-coital ache.

CAUSES

Probable causes include:

- congested pelvic veins (varicosities and congestion are reported in 91% of women with otherwise unexplained pelvic pain by Beard et al 1984)
- ovarian activity producing an excess of oestrogen that may increase vascular congestion (the mechanism is unknown, but symptoms may be relieved by suppressing ovulation) (Buck 1997)
- stress.

Characteristically, the woman who has chronic pelvic pain is one who:

- is aged 20–40 years, with a peak at 30 years
- is more likely to have had previous abdominal/pelvic surgery (Buck 1997)
- may or may not have children
- may have suffered stressful life-events, e.g:
    - bereavement, recent or in the past
    - disturbed family relationships
    - marital problems
    - employment problems
    - stressful lifestyle
    - abuse (physical, sexual or child abuse, or rape).

(Steele 1997)

INCIDENCE

The incidence of pelvic pain is as follows:

- 340 000 women in the UK

- up to 14 000 new cases each year (Davies et al 1992)
- in two-thirds of women having laparoscopy for pelvic pain no pathology will be found (Chamberlain 1995).

INVESTIGATIONS

Usual investigations for pelvic pain are:

- Careful history.
- Physical examination, which may demonstrate tenderness of the ovaries.
- Laparoscopy, which may exclude other pathology or reveal congested veins/varicosities.
- Vaginal ultrasound scan, which may:
  - exclude other pathology
  - reveal congested veins
  - demonstrate polycystic ovaries in 56% of women with pelvic pain.
- Pelvic venogram, which demonstrates dilatation, pooling and delayed clearance of contrast medium from pelvic veins – now considered too invasive for routine diagnostic use (Buck 1997).

OTHER CAUSES OF PELVIC PAIN

Gynaecological causes include:

- endometriosis
- chronic pelvic inflammatory disease
- adhesions
- fibroids
- uterovaginal prolapse
- ovarian cysts.

Non-gynaecological causes include:

- irritable bowel syndrome
- diverticular disease
- recurrent urinary tract infection
- renal calculi.

TREATMENT

Treatment will depend on the presence or absence of other pathology. If no other pathology:

- Combined oral contraceptive and NSAIDs usually have little effect.
- Medroxyprogesterone acetate for at least 3–4 months reduces pelvic blood flow by suppressing ovarian activity, if used long-term it may be necessary to 'add back' oestrogen to prevent bone loss and osteoporosis.
- Gonadotrophin releasing hormone (GnRH) analogue suppresses ovarian function; oestrogen may need to be added to counteract menopausal symptoms and possible bone loss and osteoporosis.
- Hysterectomy and bilateral salpingo-oophorectomy (in the woman who has completed her family) is considered when symptoms are very disabling.
- Psychological interventions (stress and pain management using deep relaxation techniques), combined with hormone treatment give the best long-term relief (Farquhar et al 1989).

Nursing issues

Spend some time thinking about the following:

- these women are often seen as 'heart-sink' patients and so may not get the care they merit and need (Steele 1997)
- understanding that the pain can interfere with their daily living and have a severely detrimental effect on their personal relationships
- understanding that fear of triggering the pain can stop all sexual activities
- being aware that there are specialist centres to which women can be referred
- having an understanding of the drugs that may be used
- the monthly visit for the GnRH analogue is an excellent opportunity to provide continuing psychological support
- being able to discuss alternative methods of pain relief (acupuncture, etc).

REFERENCES

Beard RW, Highman JH, Pearce S, Reginald PW 1984 Diagnosis of pelvic varicosities in women with chronic pelvic pain. Lancet ii: 946–949
Buck P 1997 Pelvic pain. In: Luesley DM (ed) Common conditions in gynaecology. Chapman & Hall Medical, London, Ch 5
Chamberlain G (ed) 1995 Sexual and reproductive health. In: Gynaecology by ten teachers, 16th edn. Edward Arnold, London, Ch 11
Davies L, Gangar KF, Drummond MS, Beard RW 1992 The economic burden of intractable gynaecological pain. British Journal of Obstetrics and Gynaecology 12 (supplement 2): 54–56

Farquhar CM, Rogers V, Franks S, Pearce S, Wadsworth J, Beard RW 1989 A randomised controlled trial of medroxyprogesterone acetate and psychotherapy for the treatment of pelvic congestion. British Journal of Obstetrics and Gynaecology 96: 1153–1162

Steele J 1997 Common gynaecological problems. In: Andrews G (ed) Women's sexual health. Baillière Tindall, London, Ch 16

Wiener J 1994. Chronic pelvic pain. The Practitioner 298: 352, 355–357

FURTHER READING

Kennedy S, Parkes J 1997 Chronic pelvic pain. In: McPherson A, Waller D (eds) Women's health, 4th edn. Oxford University Press, Oxford, Ch 15

RESOURCE

The Endometriosis Society, Suite 50, Westminister Palace Gardens, 50 Artillery Row, London SW 1P 1RL, UK. Tel.: 020 7222 2776.

CONTINENCE ISSUES

Urinary incontinence is defined by the Royal College of Physicians (1995) as: 'involuntary or inappropriate loss of urine which can be demonstrated objectively'. It is also 'women wetting themselves when they don't want to' (Jolleys 1997). Facts about urinary incontinence are shown in Box 8.6.

Box 8.6   Facts about incontinence

Urinary incontinence:
- is not a normal part of ageing
- is not an inevitable result of childbirth
- can curtail physical activity
- can affect social and sexual relationships
- is usually kept a secret.

WHY IS IT A PROBLEM?

- It may affect as many as 3 million adults (male and female) in the UK (Withnall & Crome 1997).
- Prevalence is difficult to assess since different defining criteria can be used.

- Prevalence is probably at least 14%.
- Fewer than one-third of women will consult directly about a continence problem.
- Two-thirds of women over the age of 65, suffering urinary leakage, are not receiving any help from health or social services.
- It can cause great personal and social embarrassment.
- Incidence increases with age.
- It is believed to consume 2% of health care funding (Jolleys 1997).
- It costs the NHS about £7 million a year in aids and appliances (O'Brien & Long 1995).

PREVALENCE

Prevalence of incontinence in women is shown in Table 8.2.

Table 8.2 Prevalence of incontinence in women

Living at home	
15–44 years	5–7%
45–64 years	8–15%
over 65 years	10–20%
Living in an institution	
residential home	25%
nursing home	40%
long-stay hospital	50–75%

TYPES OF INCONTINENCE

Types of urinary incontinence are described by the main symptom, the most common being:

- stress incontinence
- urge incontinence
- mixed stress and urge incontinence.

Other types include:

- overflow incontinence
- functional incontinence.

Common causes of frequency and urgency are shown in Box 8.7.

Box 8.7 Causes of frequency and urgency

Gynaecological/urological
Urinary tract infection
Detrusor instability
Bladder lesion (cancer or stones)
Inflammation (e.g. interstitial cystitis)
Fibrosis (e.g. after radiation)
Atrophy (menopause)
External pressure (e.g. pelvic mass, fibroid)
Prolapse
Pregnancy

Medical/psychological
Drugs (e.g. diuretics)
Diabetes
Neurological conditions
(e.g. multiple sclerosis)
Excessive fluid intake
Heart failure
Habit

Nursing issues

Spend some time thinking about the following:

- awareness of need for sensitivity in supporting those with continence problems
- cure rates of over 50% are reported (RCN 1997)
- specially trained nurses can achieve an improvement/cure rate of 69% (O'Brien & Long 1995)
- nurses can provide opportunities to discuss continence issues in many settings, e.g:
  - Well Woman clinic
  - family planning clinic
  - during cervical screening
  - offering dietary advice for overweight
  - baby/child health clinics
  - at post-natal checks
  - during over 75 health checks
  - in carers' groups
- encouraging all to adopt a healthy lifestyle
- knowledge of the different types of urinary incontinence and treatment options
- awareness of social issues around incontinence
- enabling patients to access appropriate services, treatment and resources
- understanding the devastating effect that incontinence can have on quality of life
- knowledge of the mechanism of continence
- knowledge of and ability to explain investigative procedures
- supporting the woman with sensitivity
- ensuring access to specialist continence nurse.

Stress incontinence

The causes of stress incontinence are:

- a weak urethral sphincter mechanism
- urine leaks as intra-abdominal pressure rises

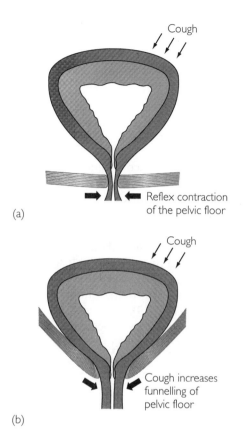

Figure 8.1 (a) Normal contraction of the pelvic floor with raised abdominal pressure. (b) Contraction of the pelvic floor with stress incontinence

- almost certainly due to weakness of the pelvic floor (Fig. 8.1)
- often provoked by coughing, sneezing or laughing
- may be provoked by even mild physical activity.

Contributory factors are shown in Box 8.8.

Treatment and management

- Accurate assessment.

Box 8.8 Contributory factors in stress incontinence

- Pregnancy and childbirth
- Menopause
- Obesity
- Chronic cough
- Lifting and straining
- Constipation.

- Differentiation of type of incontinence from symptoms, history and physical assessment.
- Advice on diet and fluid intake.
- Assessment of pelvic floor.
- 70% of women treated conservatively report being much better or cured after 12 months (Seim et al 1996).
- 75% of women treated by nurse specialists were satisfied with their quality of life (Lewey et al 1997).
- Surgery should not be considered until conservative measures have been tried (see Box 8.9).
- Urodynamic testing is not a predictor for the effectiveness of the outcome of surgery (Black et al 1997).

Box 8.9 Conservative treatment in stress incontinence

- Pelvic floor exercises
- Weighted vaginal cones
- Electrostimulation
- Oestrogen, orally or vaginally.

Urge incontinence

Urge incontinence (Cardozo & Kelleher, 1997):

- is caused by instability or hypersensitivity of the detrusor muscle (Fig. 8.2)
- the unstable bladder contracting involuntarily while filling
- is characterized by urgency, frequency and nocturia
- an underlying cause is rarely found.

Contributory factors are shown in Box 8.10.

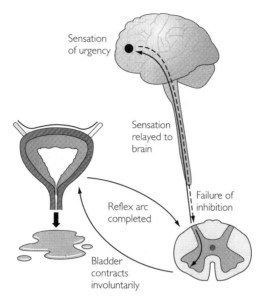

Figure 8.2   Detrusor instability (the unstable bladder).

Box 8.10   Contributory factors in urge incontinence

- Urinary tract infection
- Fluid intake
- Medication
- Anxiety.

Box 8.11   Conservative treatment for urge incontinence

- Bladder retraining (learning to pass larger volumes at longer intervals)
- Pelvic floor exercises (to strengthen the muscles)
- Electrostimulation (to restore muscle tone)
- Oestrogen replacement (when atrophic vaginitis is a contributory factor)
- Anticholinergic drugs (e.g. oxybutinin)
- Biofeedback (as part of bladder training).

Treatment and management

Conservative treatment is shown in Box 8.11. Other management is by:

- accurate assessment
- urinalysis, to exclude infection
- urodynamic assessment
- assessment of pelvic floor.

Mixed stress and urge incontinence

- Detrusor instability and stress incontinence can coexist.
- Combination of both symptoms.
- Treatment and management is by combined means.

Continence nurse specialists can carry out the following investigations:

- urinalysis
- full history
- vaginal, pelvic and abdominal examination
- bladder scan
- flow rate
- urodynamics
- assessment of perineum for signs of trauma from over-stretching during labour or from episiotomy.

The full advantages of the continence nurse specialist are set out in: *Commissioning Continence Advisory Services: An RCN Guide*, published by the Royal College of Nursing, 1997.

Vaginal cones (Dolman 1997)

- Weighted vaginal cones, of varying weight.
- Sensory feedback makes the pelvic floor contract to retain the cone in the vagina.
- The technique helps the woman to become aware of the action required to contract the pelvic floor muscle.
- Can greatly improve urinary symptoms.

Diagnostic investigations

Common investigations are:

- mid-stream urine (MSU)
- frequency/volume chart
- basic urodynamic investigation:
  - uroflowmetry (measurement of urine flow)

- cystometry (measurement of pressure/volume relationship of bladder, during filling and voiding phases)
- ultrasound to determine residual urine
- X-ray of kidney, ureters and bladder
- complex urodynamic investigation:
  - videocystourethroscopy
  - urethral pressure profile
  - electromyelography (of pelvic floor and urethral sphincter).

Surgery for stress incontinence

'The aim is to elevate the bladder neck above the level of the pelvic floor and increase urethral resistance by giving support to the urethrovesicular junction. Any co-existing uterovaginal prolapse can be corrected at the same time' (Gould 1990).

Surgical procedures (Cardozo & Kelleher 1997)

Standard surgical procedures for stress incontinence are:

- vaginal anterior colporrhaphy
- abdominal bladder neck suspensions, e.g:
  - Marshall–Marchetti–Kranz
  - Burch
  - Aldridge
- endoscopic bladder neck suspension, e.g. Stamey
- periurethral collagen injections
- artificial sphincter.

Key points

Pelvic floor exercises:

- vaginal examination usually essential for the woman to locate and contract the correct muscles
- the abdominal and gluteal muscles are not to be used
- while sitting, pretend to stop the flow of urine
- tighten the muscles and hold tight for at least 5 seconds, relax for 5 seconds; repeat five to ten times at least five times a day
- also pull up the muscles quickly for one second, relax and repeat 5 times (Dolman 1997).

Question: How long do I carry on doing my pelvic floor exercises?
Answer: Forever.

Surgery for stress incontinence is not always very successful; some post-operative problems include (Dolman 1997):

- detrusor instability
- voiding difficulties (incomplete emptying of the bladder)
- bladder pain
- dyspareunia (pain with sexual intercourse)
- failure of surgery (symptoms recurring immediately or at a later date).

REFERENCES

Black N, Griffiths J, Pope C et al 1997 Impact of surgery for stress incontinence on morbidity: cohort study. British Medical Journal 315: 1493–1498

Cardozo L, Kelleher C 1997 Problems with micturition. In: Luesley D (ed) Common conditions in gynaecology. Chapman & Hall, London, Ch 12

Dolman M 1997 Continence issues. In: Andrews G (ed) Women's sexual health. Baillière Tindall, London, Ch 15

Gould D 1990 Urinary problems. In: Gould D Nursing care of women. Prentice Hall, New York, Ch 11

Jolleys J 1997 Urinary incontinence. In: McPherson A, Waller D (eds) Women's health, 4th edn. Oxford University Press, Oxford, Ch 16

Lewey J, Billington A, O'Hara L 1997 Conservative treatment of urinary incontinence. Nursing Standard 12 (8): 45–47

O'Brien J, Long H 1995 Urinary incontinence: long term effectiveness of nursing interventions in primary care. British Medical Journal 311: 1208

Royal College of Nursing 1997 Commissioning continence advisory services: an RCN Guide. London

Royal College of Physicians' Working Party 1995 Incontinence causes, management, and provision of services. RCP, London

Seim A, Bjorg S, Eriksen B et al 1996 Treatment of urinary incontinence in women in general practice: observational study. British Medical Journal 312: 1459–1462

Withnall A and Crome P 1997 Towards better care for incontinent patients. Trends in Urology, Gynaecology and Sexual Health, September 1997: 15–16

FURTHER READING

Dolman M 1997 Continence issues. In: Andrews G (ed) Women's sexual health. Baillière Tindall, London, Ch 15

Gould D 1990 Urinary problems. In: Gould D, Nursing care of women. Prentice Hall, New York, Ch 11

Jolleys J 1997 Urinary incontinence. In: McPherson A, Waller D (eds) Women's health, 4th edn. Oxford University Press, Oxford, Ch 16

RESOURCES

Association for Continence Advice, Winchester House, Kennington Park, Cranmer Road, The Oval, London SW9 6EJ, UK. Tel.: 020 7820 8113.

The Continence Foundation, 16 Baldwin Gardens, London EC1N 7RG, UK. Tel.: 020 7404 6875.

CYSTITIS

Cystitis is inflammation of the lining of the bladder.

GENERAL FACTS
Causes

Causes of cystitis:

- 50% of the time it is caused by infection from bacteria, viruses, or fungi
- 50% of women have no demonstrable bacteriuria
- a residual pool of urine in the bladder may act as a reservoir for infection.

Significance

Cystitis is significant for the following reasons:

- At least 50% of women will experience an episode of cystitis at some time in their lives.
- 90% of these will have a single or isolated attack.
- 10% will have recurrent attacks, due to relapse or reinfection.
- Recurrent or persistent infections can result in significant kidney damage (Baker & Tomson 1994).
- In the UK 1–3% of all consultations to general practitioners (GPs) are for urinary tract infections (Hope 1997).

Symptoms

General symptoms of cystitis:

- frequency of micturition by day and night
- dysuria, often called burning or scalding
- suprapubic pain or tenderness
- haematuria
- smelly urine.

BACTERIAL CYSTITIS

Women are susceptible to ascending infection because of the short, straight female urethra.

- 85% of cystitis is caused by Escherichia coli.
- Less common pathogens are *Proteus* and *Klebsiella.*
- Rarely, the organism may be *Chlamydia* or genital herpes.

Bowel flora can contaminate the urethra in the following ways:

- poor personal hygiene leaving the perineum contaminated
- by not wiping from 'front to back'
- sanitary towels and tight-fitting trousers can massage the bacteria along the perineum to the urethra
- during sexual intercourse
- while inserting vaginal tampons.

The reduction in lactobacilli in the vagina of the post-menopausal woman allows the pH of the vagina to rise, combined with atrophy of the vaginal and urethral mucosa, colonization with pathogens is much more likely.

NON-BACTERIAL CYSTITIS

Symptoms of frequency and dysuria, in the absence of bacteria, indicate a non-bacterial cause of cystitis. Also called the 'urethral syndrome'.

Causes

Some possible causes:

- constipation and ill-fitting contraceptive diaphragms can delay bladder emptying
- vaginal tampon may delay bladder emptying
- sexual activity, causing irritation to the posterior bladder wall
- caffeine (contained in tea, coffee and cola drinks) can excite the detrusor muscle in the bladder
- atrophic vaginitis or urethritis in the post-menopausal woman
- vaginitis and urethritis caused by STIs
- chemical contamination from soaps, bubble bath, detergent, spermicide, deodorant, antiseptics
- inadequate fluid intake

- infrequent and inadequate bladder emptying
- possible allergic response to some spiced foods, refined foods and citrus fruits
- interstitial cystitis.

Nursing issues

Spend some time thinking about the following:

- encouraging a lifestyle that will reduce the risk of infection (e.g. personal hygiene)
- identifying those at risk of cystitis e.g:
  - previous episode of infection
  - in a first or new sexual relationship
  - menopausal and post-menopausal women
- awareness of opportunities to discuss issues e.g:
  - health education in schools
  - consulation around contraception
  - visit for cervical smear
  - discussion about menopause
  - elderly health check (disability can make it difficult to maintain personal hygeine)
- knowledge of measures to help prevent reinfection and recurrence
- awareness of the impact that recurrent cystitis can have on a woman's life, well-being and relationships
- knowledge of local and national resources and information
- awareness of referral criteria for specialist advice.

Key points

- Loin pain, low back pain, pyrexia and systemic upset suggest an upper urinary tract infection.
- One-third of characteristic cases of acute cystitis have an unrecognized infection of the upper urinary tract (Hope 1997).
- There are a number of risk factors for upper urinary tract infection and consequent kidney damage:
  - diabetes mellitus
  - pregnancy
  - urinary tract abnormality
  - urinary stone.
- Bladder urine is sterile with pH range 4.3–7.25.
- *E. coli* thrives in pH 6.0–7.0.
- Low urine pH <5 decreases the ability of *E. coli* to multiply.
- Some consider the dipstick test for nitrites has an unacceptably high false-negative detection rate.
- Contamination and delay in transporting the sample can significantly affect the value of the findings.
- Trimethoprin does not usually affect the flora of the bowel and urethra, so a woman is unlikely to be affected by *Candida albicans* (thrush) (see p. 159) following treatment.

INTERSTITIAL CYSTITIS

Interstitial cystitis facts:

- uncommon, very painful condition of unknown cause
- possibly caused by an autoimmune disorder
- cystoscopy demonstrates inflammatory changes with ulceration of the bladder base
- frequency, dysuria and severe suprapubic pain
- woman almost always aged over 40 years
- sterile urine
- treatments include oral steroids, bladder instillation with a NSAID and bladder stretching
- symptoms can be so severe and disabling that a woman may contemplate cystectomy as a remedy.

MANAGEMENT
Diagnosis

- Accurate and sensitive history, noting any changes in lifestyle or sexual activity.
- Dipstick for presence of leucocytes and nitrites.
- Urine sample to laboratory for culture and sensitivity.

Treatment

Treatment is either by antibiotics or self-help methods.

Antibiotics

Antibiotics can be started before the results of the urine culture are known. The antibiotic of choice is trimethoprin (contraindicated in pregnancy and severe renal disease, caution with breast feeding). Other recommended antibiotics include:

- amoxycillin
- nitrofurantoin (contraindicated in impaired renal function, pregnancy at term and breast-feeding).

Self-help

Managing an attack of cystitis:

- drink half a pint of water every 20 minutes for 3 hours
- alkalinize the urine with one teaspoon of bicarbonate of soda in water, potassium citrate or other alkalinizing agents (caution in those with renal impairment or cardiac disease, or who are pregnant); this can relieve the discomfort
- regularly take preferred analgesics
- put one hot water bottle in the small of the back and another, wrapped in a towel, high up between the legs
- it may be less painful to pass urine while sitting in a warm bath.

REFERENCES

Baker LRI, Tomson CRV 1994 Renal disease. In: Kumar P, Clark M (eds) Clinical medicine, 3rd edn. Saunders, London, Ch 9
Hope S 1997 Cystitis. In: McPherson A, Waller D (eds) Women's health, 4th edn. Oxford University Press, Oxford, Ch 14

FURTHER READING

Clayton C 1995 Coping with cystitis. Sheldon Press, London
Hope S 1997 Cystitis. In: McPherson A, Waller D (eds) Women's health. Oxford University Press, Oxford, Ch 14
Kilmartin A 1994 Cystitis: how to prevent infection and inflammation. Thorsons, London

RESOURCES

Health Education Authority (leaflets), 30 Great Peter Street, London SW1 9RT, UK. Tel.: 020 7222 5300.

Women's Health Concern (leaflets), PO Box 1629, London SW15 2ZL, UK. Tel: 020 8780 3916.

DYSMENORRHOEA

Dysmenorrhoea is pain associated with menstruation, and is usually described as primary or secondary. **Primary dysmenorrhoea** is now defined as pain with menstruation in the absence of evident pelvic disease; **secondary dysmenorrhoea** being pain with menstruation due to evident pelvic disease (Chamberlain 1995).

PRIMARY DYSMENORRHOEA

Primary dysmenorrhoea:

- is the more common
- does not usually occur in anovulatory cycles
- usually occurs once regular ovulatory cycles are established
- starts around the onset of bleeding, usually lasting one to two days
- is common in girls and young women (15–25 years)
- the pain is colicky, sometimes settling to a dull ache
- the pain may be accompanied by:
  - backache
  - nausea/vomiting
  - diarrhoea
  - faintness
- the pain can be severe enough for a young woman to attend an A&E department as an emergency
- pelvic examination is normal.

Incidence

At least 75% of women will have painful periods at some time in their lives. Between 5 and 15% of young women are incapacitated every month (Bowen-Simpkins 1996).

Causes

Dysmenorrhoea is probably due to an excess production of prostaglandin from the endometrium, which promotes intense uterine contractions. Prostaglandins cause spasm of the myometrium and necrosis of the endometrium. Rarely it is caused by congenital abnormality of the genital tract.

Management

Management will depend on:
- age
- severity of symptoms
- contraceptive needs
- own wishes.

NSAIDs are prostaglandin synthetase inhibitors and can be very effective, taken at the onset of menstruation. For example:

- aspirin
- mefenamic acid
- ibuprofen
- naproxen
- indomethacin.

Paracetomol may be better tolerated by some women.

The combined oral contraceptive (COC) can be highly effective, by suppressing ovulation. Anovulatory cycles are associated with a reduction in the capacity of the endometrium to produce prostaglandins. Progestogen may help where the COC is contraindicated: dydrogesterone, from days 5 to 25 of the cycle.

Nursing issues

Spend some time thinking about the following:

- acknoledgment of the pain and fear
- awareness of traditional, usually male, response of dismissing the pain as being 'all in the mind' and of hysterical origin
- knowledge of social and cultural expectations of menstruation
- awareness that there can be highly negative expectations of menstruation
- discussing possible causes
- providing information on self-help e.g: .
  - diet (to prevent constipation)
  - exercise (encourages to release of endogenous endorphins)
  - heat (hot water bottle or heated pad to pelvic/back area)
  - stress releif (by learning relaxation techniques)
- ensuring adequate pain relief (see p. 283)
- understanding the difference between the two types of dysmenorrhoea, so that the appropriate treatment and care can be given.

SECONDARY DYSMENORRHOEA

Secondary dysmenorrhoea:

- affects older women (over 25 years usually)
- pain often starts before the onset of bleeding (may be up one week)

Key points

Any woman who has severe dysmenorrhoea that is not relieved by any treatment should be referred for a specialist opinion:

- there may be pelvic pathology
- she may respond to more aggressive treatment
- dilatation and curettage (D&C) used to be regularly carried out; there is no research evidence that this is clinically effective.

- pelvic pathology is present e.g:
  - pelvic inflammatory disease
  - endometriosis
  - submucosal fibroid
- may be caused by intrauterine contraceptive device (IUD).

Investigations are carried out to determine cause. Treatment is according to cause, as appropriate.

REFERENCES

Bowen-Simpkins P 1996 Primary dysmenorrhoea: causes and treatment. Prescriber, 5 August: 23, 24, 28, 29, 30, 34, 35, 37–39
Chamberlain G (ed) 1995 Menstrual disorders. In: Gynaecology by ten teachers, 16th edn. Arnold, London, Ch 8

ENDOMETRIAL CANCER

Endometrial cancer is a cancer originating in the endometrium, that is, the lining of the uterus. It may also be referred to as cancer of the uterus or uterine cancer. It is nearly always an adenocarcinoma. Endometrial hyperplasia can be a precursor to endometrial cancer. Endometrial cancer is less common than cervical cancer (see p. 259), and is most commonly seen in the post-menopausal woman.

CAUSES

It is probably caused by excessive exposure of the endometrium to oestrogen. This may be due to (Redman 1997):

- obesity – adipose tissue converts increased amounts of androstenedione into oestrone (a post-menopausal oestrogen)
- late menopause
- unopposed oestrogen – as hormone replacement therapy (HRT) in the woman who has not had a hysterectomy (see p. 176)
- anovulatory menstrual cycles:
  - these tend to occur close to the menopause
  - or as in polycystic ovary syndrome (PCOS) (see p. 318)
- oestrogen-secreting ovarian tumours.

Risk factors

Associated risk factors are:

- age – mean incidence is 60 years
- nulliparity
- infertility
- family history – more common in families in which other members have breast or bowel cancer
- higher socio-economic status.

SYMPTOMS

Symptoms are:

- irregular heavy periods
- intermenstrual bleeding
- post-menopausal bleeding (the most common symptom)
- postcoital bleeding (bleeding after sexual intercourse).

DIAGNOSIS

Diagnosis is by endometrial sampling for histological examination. It is usually carried out in gynaecological clinics, and has significantly reduced the number of inpatient stays for traditional dilation and curettage (D&C) (Cassidy 1997).

An ultrasound scan can demonstrate the thickness of the endometrium and the presence of any uterine abnormality, e.g. fibroid or endometrial polyps. It does not replace biopsy for diagnosis.

Hysteroscopy is where a hysteroscope is passed through the cervix, for inspection and for sampling of the endometrium for histological examination. It can be carried out under local or general anaesthetic.

TREATMENT

Treatment is usually surgery (probably removal of the uterus, uterine tubes and ovaries) and radiotherapy, either before or after the surgery. Hormonal treatment and chemotherapy may also be used.

Treatment will depend on:

- the woman's age
- her general health
- the type and extent of the tumour.

Nursing issues

Spend some time thinking about the following:

- awareness of the incidence of endometrial cancer
- understanding the importance of early diagnosis and treatment
- knowledge of some of the treatment and management options available locally
- ensuring that all post-menopausal women understand the importance of reporting any bleeding that is not associated with taking HRT
- understanding the importance of monitoring the bleeding pattern of women who are taking HRT
- encouraging attendance for routine cervical screening, which should be an opportunity for voicing any concerns
- awareness of the distress caused by a diagnosis of cancer
- awareness of the effects on the woman's sexuality and relationships
- awareness that some women have not completed their childbearing.

Key points

- The frequency of endometrial cancer is reduced in users of the contraceptive-pill (COC) (see p. 115):
  - the incidence is halved among all users
  - is reduced to one third in long-term users
  - the protective effect can be detected in ex-users for 10–15 years (Guillebaud 1997).
- Post-menopausal bleeding should be regarded as cancer until proven otherwise (Redman 1997).
- 75% of endometrial cancers occur in the post-menopausal period
  - 5% will develop before the age of 40
  - a further 20% develop before the menopause (Chamberlain 1995).
- Twenty per cent of women with post-menopausal bleeding will have a genital tract malignancy (Chamberlain 1995).
- Age alone should not be considered as a contraindication to surgical management.
- Many elderly women can be fit to tolerate radical surgery (Redman 1997).

REFERENCES

Cassidy L 1997 The gynaecological examination. In: Luesley D (ed) Common conditions in gynaecology. Chapman & Hall, London, Ch 2

Chamberlain G (ed) 1995 Gynaecological tumors. In: Gynaecology by ten teachers, 16th edn. Arnold, London, Ch 6

Guillebaud J 1997 Contraception. In: McPherson A, Waller D (eds) Women's health, 4th edn. Oxford University Press, Oxford, Ch 6

Redman C 1997 Gynaecological cancers. In: Luesley D (ed) Common conditions in gynaecology. Chapman & Hall, London, Ch 10

FURTHER READING

CancerBACUP Understanding cancer of the uterus and Sexuality and cancer

RESOURCES

CancerBACUP, 3 Bath Place, Rivington Street, London EC2A 3JR, UK.

Cancer Information Service, Tel: 020 7613 2121. Freeline (for calls from outside London) 0800 18 11 99.

ENDOMETRIOSIS

Endometriosis is one of the most common benign gynaecological conditions. It may be defined as the presence of functioning endometrial glands outside their usual location lining the uterine cavity (Rock & Markham 1992). Endometriosis is the proliferation of endometrial tissue in sites other than the uterine mucosa (Fig. 8.3); if the deposit is within the myometrium it is known as *adenomyosis*.

The endometriotic sites may occur anywhere in the pelvis, mainly affecting the ovaries, uterine tubes, the pelvic peritoneum, the rectovaginal pouch and the uterosacral ligaments. Deposits have been found throughout the pelvis, including in the bowel, bladder, cervix, vagina and vulva. Deposits have been reported as far away as the pleura.

WHY IT IS A PROBLEM

- Because ectopic endometrial tissue responds to the hormonal fluctuations of the menstrual cycle, bleeding may occur at the site of the deposit.
- In the ovary the bleeding may result in a 'chocolate cyst' (a cyst filled with old blood).
- Adhesions form around endometriotic lesions, affecting uterus, adnexa (uterine tubes and ovaries), bowel and omentum.
- Endometriosis can affect fertility.

WHY IT HAPPENS

There are a number of theories as to the aetiology:

- Retrograde menstruation: the flow of menstrual blood backward through the uterine tubes rather than forward through the cervix (this is considered the most likely).
- Lymphatic or vascular transportation.

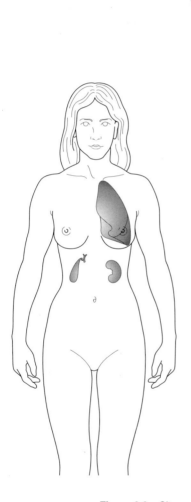

Figure 8.3 Sites of endometriosis.

- Embryological migration (misplacing of peritoneal endothelial cells during embryological development).
- Transfer of cells during surgery (e.g. hysterotomy).
- An autoimmune response.

SYMPTOMS

Many of the symptoms are cyclical, being aggravated by menstruation. However, other symptoms, particularly dyspareunia (pain with sexual intercourse), may be present the whole time, since the uterus may become fixed in retroversion and there can be tender masses in the rectovaginal septum. Symptoms will depend on which organs are involved.

Common symptoms

Common symptoms include:

- dysmenorrhoea
- dyspareunia
- menorrhagia
- infertility
- irregular uterine bleeding
- rectal pain
- pain on defecation.

Less common symptoms

Less common symptoms include:

- frequency of micturition and dysuria
- cyclical haematuria
- cyclical rectal bleeding
- bowel obstruction
- cyclical haemoptysis.

Cyclical symptoms occur at the time of the menstrual period.

INCIDENCE

- There is no consensus as to the incidence, but it could be in excess of 10% of women.

Nursing issues

Spend some time thinking about the following:

- helping the woman describe her symptoms as accurately as possible
- some women have been labelled 'neurotic' before a diagnosis has been made
- mild disease can still produce severe symptoms
- understanding fears for future fertility
- symptoms, especially dyspareunia, can precipitate relationship difficulties
- being able to explain any surgical or invasive procedure
- understanding and being able to explain the drug therapies, including side-effects, contraindications and any special precautions (e.g. the risk of danazol having a masculinizing effect on a female fetus)
- supplying educational literature
- supplying information re support groups.

- It is most common in the reproductive years, particularly in women who delay pregnancy.
- It is much more common in first degree relatives of women with endometriosis.
- The disease usually regresses at the menopause.

DIAGNOSIS

- Initially by pelvic examination and pelvic ultrasound, which may demonstrate ovarian cysts.
- Laparoscopy is essential for differential diagnosis.
- Laparoscopic examination can identify the characteristic 'powder burn' appearance of the endometriotic lesions and/or 'chocolate' cysts; the lesions may be too few and far between to be visualized.

Powder burn lesions look like the marks left by cigarette burns; chocolate cysts are so called because they contain altered blood that resembles chocolate.

ENDOMETRIOSIS AND INFERTILITY

- There appears to be an association, since 30–70% of women investigated for infertility are found to have endometriosis in varying degrees of severity (Kennedy 1993).
- The relationship between the two is thought to relate to multiple factors: ovarian function, tubal function, peritoneal environment and altered immunity (Rock & Markham 1992).

- There can be gross distortion of the pelvic organs in severe disease.
- Tubal damage is secondary to adhesions rather than primary endometriotic deposits (Buck 1997).

Endometriosis may be found in 'normal' women having laparoscopy for other reasons.

TREATMENT

The aims of treatment are:

- to relieve symptoms
- to limit the disease
- to preserve fertility (if wanted by the woman).

The treatment will depend on:

- the extent of the disease
- the severity of the symptoms
- the woman's age
- the woman's desire for a future pregnancy
- the woman's wishes.

Treatment can be medical or surgical, or a combination of the two.

Medical treatments

NSAIDs have an anti-prostaglandin effect (prostaglandins produce vasoconstriction and uterine contractions); for example, mefenamic acid and naproxen. Nausea and gastrointestinal disturbance are the most common adverse effects of these drugs. Pseudopregnancy drugs suppress ovulation, e.g. combined oestrogen and progestogen (30 µg COC given continuously for 4–6 months) or progestogens (dydrogesterone 10–30 mg daily) or medroxyprogesterone acetate (10 mg three times daily).

Treatment should be reviewed at six months.

Possible side-effects are:

- fluid retention
- nausea
- breast tenderness
- breakthrough bleeding
- other premenstrual-type symptoms.

Androgen, decreasing gonadotropin releasing hormone (GnRH) and inhibiting luteinizing hormone (LH) can also be used, e.g. danazol 200 mg three times daily for up to six months. This drug is less frequently used, owing to its considerable side-effects, however it can be a very effective treatment.

Possible side-effects are:

- weight gain
- mood swings
- depression
- acne
- reduction in sex drive
- muscle cramps
- hot sweats
- oily skin
- effect on lipoprotein metabolism
- hirsutism
- headaches
- voice change (rare).

Pseudomenopause or suppression of ovarian activity can be brought about by e.g. GnRH analogues:

- buserelin nasal spray 150 µg into each nostril three times daily
- nafarelin nasal spray 200 µg twice daily
- goserelin 3.6 mg implant into anterior abdominal wall every 28 days
- leuprorelin 3.75 s.c. or i.m injection every 28 days.

Side-effects are menopausal symptoms or probable loss of bone density after six months' use. Medical treatment can have a dramatic effect on symptoms, but they often return after treatment has stopped (Buck 1997).

Alternative therapies: evening primrose oil (containing gamolenic acid, GLA) can relieve:

- breast pain
- abdominal pain
- mood swings.

It is believed that GLA corrects a theoretical disorder between prostaglandins and essential fatty acids. These symptoms may be related to medical treatment (Hawkridge 1989).

Other recommended treatments include: vitamin E, vitamin C, selenium, magnesium, calcium and zinc. However there is no rigorous research to support these theories.

Surgical treatment

Conservative surgery aims to restore normal pelvic anatomy and eliminate active disease using laparoscopy to carry out:

- diathermy
- laser
- microsurgery
- enucleation of chocolate cysts.

Radical surgery can be hysterectomy and bilateral salpingo-oophorectomy, together with HRT (Shaw 1992).

Key points

- Other conditions can have similar signs and symptoms as endometriosis and should be excluded:
  - pelvic inflammatory disease
  - ectopic pregnancy
  - ovarian cysts
  - urinary tract infection.
- There is no correlation between severity of disease and severity of symptoms.
- Treatment with HRT following radical surgery does not appear to be associated with recurrence of disease (Chamberlain 1995).

REFERENCES

Buck P 1997 Pelvic pain. In: Luesley DM (ed) Common conditions in gynaecology. Chapman & Hall Medical, London, Ch 5
Chamberlain G (ed) 1995 Gynaecology by ten teachers, 16th edn. Arnold, London, Ch 7
Hawkridge C 1989 Understanding endometriosis. Optima, London
Kennedy S 1993 Endometriosis. In: Women's problems in general practice, 3rd edn. Oxford University Press, Oxford, Ch 12
Rock JA, Markham SM 1992 Pathogenesis of endometriosis. Lancet 340: 1264–1267
Shaw RW 1992 Treatment of endometriosis. Lancet 340: 1267–1271

FURTHER READING

Mears J 1996 Coping with endometriosis. Sheldon, London

RESOURCES

National Endometriosis Society (self-help group and information), 50 Westminster Palace Gardens, Artillery Row, London SW1 1RL, UK. Tel.: 020 222 2781.

The Publications Office (leaflets)

Royal College of Obstetricians and Gynaecologists, 27 Sussex Place, Regent's Park, London NW1 4RG, UK. Tel.: 020 7262 5425.

Women's Health Concern (leaflets and information), PO Box 1629, London SW15 2ZL, UK. Tel.: 020 8780 3916.

FIBROIDS

Uterine fibroids, or *leiomyomata*, are benign tumours arising in the myometrium (Fig. 8.4). They are the commonest gynaecological disorder, affecting 20–25% of women aged over 35 years (Rees 1997) and are three times more common in women of Afro-Caribbean descent than white women (Chamberlain 1995): the reason for this is not known.

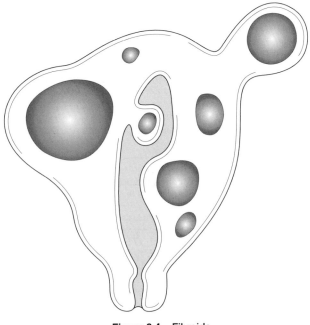

Figure 8.4   Fibroids

Fibroids are composed of smooth muscle and fibrous tissue and are described by their location:

- submucosal (beneath the endometrium)
- subserosal (under the peritoneum of the uterus)
- intramural (within the muscle of the uterus)
- cervical (around 2%).

Fibroids can be single or multiple, may become pedunculated, or polypoid, and are probably oestrogen dependent, since they regress after the menopause. They generally grow slowly; 0.2% of fibroids may become malignant, to form a sarcoma.

EFFECTS

Regardless of size and number, many women will be asymptomatic. The most common symptom is menorrhagia (excessive menstrual bleeding), possibly caused by a submucosal fibroid protruding into the uterine cavity and increasing the surface area of the endometrium to be shed at a period. Periods are usually still regular.

Other symptoms will depend on the size and location of the fibroid; large ones may press on surrounding organs:

- bladder, causing frequency or retention
- bowel, causing constipation
- hugely enlarging the uterus, causing abdominal distension.

Women can be asymptomatic even with a huge fibroid, which may be found coincidently.

FERTILITY

Fibroids can affect fertility:

- pregnancy is less likely if the fibroid is submucosal
- miscarriage is more likely if the fibroid is submucosal or intramural
- the uterine cavity can be grossly distorted
- the uterine tubes can be distorted
- labour may be obstructed.

PAIN

Pain is not usually a symptom of fibroids, but could be caused by:

- torsion of a pedunculated fibroid
- degeneration of a fibroid
- stretching of the peritoneum by a rapidly growing fibroid (Buck 1997)
- infection of a fibroid after delivery or abortion
- sarcomatous change (Chamberlain 1995).

DIAGNOSIS

Pelvic examination will usually confirm the presence of fibroids. However, pelvic ultrasound will reveal the:

- size
- number
- location
- type.

Ultrasound examination will give a differential diagnosis, since menorrhagia can be caused by other conditions, such as:

- adenomyosis
- endometriosis
- pelvic inflammatory disease
- intrauterine contraceptive device
- ovarian tumours and cysts
- other pelvic or uterine cancers.

TREATMENT

Treatment will depend on the woman's:

- symptoms
- age, with regard to maintaining fertility
- own wishes.

Medical treatment

Drugs or devices may be used to reduce the amount of blood loss or to reduce the size of the fibroids such as:

- prostaglandin synthetase inhibitors
- antifibrinolytics
- progestogens
- combined oral contraceptive

- androgenic preparations
- intrauterine system (IUS) (West 1992).

An example of a prostaglandin synthetase inhibitor is mefenamic acid (Ponstan) 500 mg three times a day starting on the first day of menstrual bleeding. This drug is not as effective as was once thought in reducing blood loss (NB it may cause diarrhoea).

An example of an antifibrinolytic is tranexamic acid (Cyklokapron) 1–1.5 g three to four times a day. Start with heavy bleeding and take for 3–4 days (NB it may cause gastrointestinal upset and increase risk of thrombosis).

Progestogens used can be: norethisterone 5 mg three times a day for 10 days to arrest bleeding or from day 19 to day 26 of the cycle to prevent bleeding (NB possible nausea, exacerbation of migraine and epilepsy) or medroxyprogesterone acetate 2.5–10 mg daily for 5–10 days, beginning on 16th–21st day of cycle and repeating for two to three cycles (NB may cause androgenic side-effects).

Surgical treatment

Surgical options are:

- myomectomy ('shelling out' of fibroid), via
  - abdomen
  - vagina
  - endoscope
- hysterectomy
  - vaginal
  - abdominal

Nursing issues

Spend some time thinking about the following:

- ensuring a good knowledge of all treatment options
- respecting the woman's choice of treatment
- is the woman anaemic or hypothyroid?
- having a knowledge of the action, indications, contraindications, precautions and side-effects of drugs used
- having an understanding of the concerns and anxieties of the woman who has not started or completed her child-bearing
- some women believe that a diet that is low in 'natural' oestrogens (i.e. plant or phyto-oestrogens) will improve their symptoms. There is no evidence to support this belief.

Key points

- If there is irregular bleeding another diagnosis should be suspected and investigated.
- It is essential for the woman to be involved in decisions about her treatment:
  - only the woman knows how tolerable or otherwise her symptoms are
  - there may be racism in the treatment of women with fibroids: Afro-Caribbean women feel that they are not given the treatment options that white women are given, and are only offered hysterectomy (Douglas 1998).

REFERENCES

Buck P 1997 Pelvic pain. In: Luesley DM (ed) Common conditions in gynaecology. Chapman & Hall, London, Ch 5
Chamberlain G (ed) 1995 Gynaecological tumours. In: Gynaecology by ten teachers, 16th edn. Arnold, London, Ch 6
Douglas J 1998 Meeting the health needs of women from black and minority ethnic communities. In: Doyal L (ed) Women and health services. Open University Press, Buckingham, Ch 4
Rees M 1997. Menstrual problems. In: McPherson A, Waller D (eds) Women's health, 4th edn. Oxford University Press, Oxford, Ch 10
West C 1992 Management of uterine fibroids. The Practitioner 236: 117–119

GENITAL PROLAPSE

Genital prolapse is:

- the displacement of one or more of the pelvic organs
- displacement is downward, through the vagina
- the uterus is the most commonly affected organ
- the bladder, urethra and rectum can also prolapse into the vagina
- it is a very common condition
- is more likely to occur in older women
- prolapse and prolapse-related problems account for nearly a quarter of women waiting for routine gynecological surgery (Creighton & Lawton 1997).

CAUSES

It is caused by weakness of the muscles and ligaments of the pelvic floor. The weakness may be caused by (Creighton & Lawton 1997):

- Childbirth:
  - this is the most common reason
  - muscles and ligaments can be over-stretched during vaginal delivery (particularly if there is a long second stage of labour or a very large baby)
  - there may be problems immediately after delivery, but they more commonly present in later life.
- Collagen abnormality:
  - this may explain why some nulliparous women develop prolapse
  - and why some multiparous women do not develop prolapse
  - and why it is rare in Afro-Caribbean women.
- Hormonal status:
  - prolapse is more common after the menopause
  - low oestrogen levels may result in weakening and atrophy of the muscles and ligaments
  - there is no evidence that giving HRT (see p. 176) reduces the incidence of prolapse.
- Raised intra-abdominal pressure:
  - persistent cough (e.g. in smoker)
  - chronic constipation
  - obesity
  - large pelvic mass (e.g. large fibroid) (see p. 294).
- Previous pelvic surgery:
  - abdominal and vaginal hysterectomy may predispose to the development of prolapse
  - a repair operation to the anterior wall of the vagina for stress incontinence may predispose to a prolapse of the posterior vaginal wall.

TYPES OF PROLAPSE

Uterine

The uterus descends through the vagina.

- 1st degree – the cervix does not reach the introitus (the entrance to the vagina).
- 2nd degree – the cervix can be seen at the introitus.
- 3rd degree – the cervix and uterus have prolapsed through the introitus (also called procidentia).

Vaginal wall

Type of prolapse depends on the structure directly adjacent:

- *cystocele* – prolapse of upper part of the anterior vaginal wall, contains bladder.
- *urethrocele* – lower part of anterior vaginal wall, contains urethra.
- *rectocele* – middle part of posterior vaginal wall, contains rectum.
- *enterocele* – upper part of posterior vaginal wall, adjacent to rectovaginal pouch, contains small bowel or omentum.

SYMPTOMS

- A dragging sensation, a feeling of 'something coming down' or a bulging lump in the vagina are the most commonly reported symptoms.
- Backache, that is worse on standing and is relieved by lying down.
- Urinary symptoms:
  - frequency and dysuria, caused by incomplete emptying of the bladder
  - stress incontinence (see p. 268).
- Bowel symptoms – pain or difficulty with defaecation.
- Dyspareunia – pain or difficulty with sexual intercourse.
- Many women do not recognize that they have a problem, putting symptoms down to 'wear and tear' or 'old age'.

TREATMENT

Treatment depends on a number of factors, including:

- the severity and type of symptoms
- the possible affects on sexual relationships
- whether the woman has completed her family
- whether she is elderly, unfit or has other medical problems
- what the expected outcomes are of any treatment
- what the woman wants to do.

Conservative treatment

- Pelvic floor exercises (may help with stress incontinence).

- Supporting the prolapse with a vaginal pessary – usually a ring pessary – which must be changed every 3–6 months.

Surgical treatment

There are many different repair operations, the choice depends on the type and degree of prolapse. Uterine prolapse is usually treated by vaginal hysterectomy. Recurrent prolapse is common (Creighton & Lawton 1997).

Nursing issues

Spend some time thinking about the following:

- awareness of the incidence of genital prolapse
- understanding the need for sensitivity when discussing the symptoms
- understanding the importance of promoting and supporting strategies that will not cure the condition, but will improve the woman's health status and may make surgery easier to perform (e.g. losing weight, stopping smoking) (Creighton & Lawton 1997)
- understanding the fear that many women have at finding a 'lump' in their vagina
- knowledge of treatment and management options
- awareness of the need to respect any woman's reluctance to undergo surgery
- awareness of the impact that her symptoms may have on her family, social and sexual relationships.

Key points

- When the uterus prolapses the vagina always descends with it.
- Vaginal prolapse may occur without uterine descent (Gould 1990).
- Prevention of prolapse must be the aim, through encouraging a lifelong commitment to pelvic floor exercises for all (see p. 275).
- Frequent pregnancies at unduly short intervals may increase the risk of prolapse, partly because of the strain of lifting and carrying a baby while pregnant with the next child (Chamberlain 1995).

REFERENCES

Chamberlain G (ed) Mechanical problems. In: Gynaecology by ten teachers, 16th edn. Arnold, London, Ch 4

Creighton S, Lawton F 1997 Uterovaginal prolapse. In: Luesley D (ed) Common conditions in gynaecology. Chapman & Hall, London, Ch 11

Gould D 1990 Pelvic support. In: Gould D, Nursing care of women. Prentice Hall, New York, Ch 10

MENORRHAGIA

Menorrhagia is excessive regular menstrual blood loss.

The average menstrual blood loss is 30–40 ml and in 90% of women the loss is less than 80 ml. The widely accepted definition of menorrhagia is blood loss of 80 ml or more per menstrual cycle (Coulter et al 1995).

WHY IT IS A PROBLEM

- Less than 31% of women may describe their blood loss as heavy.
- It is one of the most common reasons for gynaecological referral.
- Many women who seek treatment for heavy bleeding in reality do not have higher than average loss (Coulter at al 1995).
- Each year around £7 million is spent in the UK on primary care prescribing on a wide variety of drugs to treat menorrhagia (Sheldon 1995).
- Five per cent of women aged 30–49 consult their GP for menorrhagia in any one year (Rees 1997).
- Women report that menorrhagia causes moodiness or irritability, depression, spoils their sex lives, and interferes with life in general.
- The condition can have a serious impact on a woman's quality of life (Coulter 1997).

CAUSES

Among the causes are:

- fibroids (see p. 294)
- endometriosis (see p. 287)
- adenomyosis (endometrial deposits within the myometrium)
- endometrial hyperplasia (which can be a precursor to endometrial cancer)
- endometrial polyps
- hypothyroidism
- chronic pelvic inflammatory disease (see p 314)
- IUD (see p. 118)

- coagulation disorder
- endometrial cancer
- cervical cancer
- cervical polyps.

Dysfunctional uterine bleeding is abnormal menstrual bleeding in the absence of any pathology. It may be due to:

- anovulatory cycles (which tend to occur soon after menarche and/or close to the menopause) in which the endometrium becomes much thicker than normal
- in ovulatory cycles, with disordered prostaglandin or fibrinolytic function.

TREATMENT AND MANAGEMENT
Guidelines

(From Effective Health Care 1995.)

What are effective ways of treating excessive regular menstrual blood loss in primary and secondary care?

- Menorrhagia accounts for a significant proportion of gynaecological referrals and over half of all hysterectomies.
- A large proportion of women who complain of heavy periods and who receive treatment have menstrual blood loss within the normal range.
- Diagnostic dilatation and curettage (D&C) should not be performed on women aged under 40 and its use in older women could be replaced by cheaper and safer methods of endometrial sampling.
- Norethisterone is one of the most commonly prescribed drugs for menorrhagia, and is possibly the least effective.
- Evidence suggests that tranexamic acid and mefenamic acid are among the most effective and acceptable of first-line treatments (O'Brien & Doyle 1997).
- The hormone-releasing intrauterine device (IUS, see p. 118) appears to be highly effective but is not yet licensed for use in menorrhagia.
- Endometrial resection and laser ablation are cheaper than hysterectomy and generally effective in the short-term; however a significant proportion of women require further surgery on one or more occasions.

- Surgeons must have the necessary training and skills before using less invasive surgical techniques, such as endometrial resection and laser ablation.
- Women report high levels of satisfaction with hysterectomy which is totally effective; however, it is more expensive and involves a longer recovery period.
- Since no one management plan is better in all respects, women should be assisted to make informed choices about how they want to be treated.
- Research is needed to compare the relative effectiveness and cost-effectiveness of the most promising form of intervention, in terms of blood loss, quality of life and patient acceptability.

Concerns about excessive bleeding

- Excessive blood loss may be sufficient to cause iron deficiency and anaemia.
- Menstrual loss escaping in gushes can be sufficient to cause soiling or saturation of clothes, and social embarrassment.
- Perceived increase in menstrual loss can lead to a fear of possible underlying cancer (Fraser 1997).

Diagnosis

Diagnosis is by:

- history
- pelvic examination
- pelvic ultrasound
- hysteroscopy
- endometrial sampling (this has largely replaced D&C as an aid to diagnosis).

Treatment summary

Treatment and management will depend on:

- the severity of the symptoms
- the nature of any underlying pathology
- the coexistence of any other problems
- the woman's desire for pregnancy, her age and her personal wishes (O'Brien & Doyle 1997).

Medical treatments

Hormonal therapies

- Progestogens
- oestrogen/progestogen
- IUS
- danazol
- gestrinone
- GnRH analogues.

Non-hormonal

- Prostaglandin synthetase inhibitors (mefenamic acid, naproxen, ibuprofen)
- antifibrinolytics (tranexamic acid)
- ethamsylate (a haemostatic agent).

Surgical treatment

Surgical treatments are hysterectomy or endometrial ablation (destruction of the endometrium) carried out by various techniques.

Nursing issues

Spend some time thinking about the following:

- awareness of the incidence of menorrhagia
- knowledge of the physiology of menstruation and of the pathology most commonly associated with menorrhagia
- offering respect and acceptance of the individual's experience and perception of menorrhagia
- awareness of the fear of underlying sinister pathology
- awareness of the impact of menorrhagia on the quality of life for any woman
- awareness of the impact of menorrhagia on the cultural or religious aspect of some women's lives
- ability to offer reliable information on the diagnosis and treatment options.

Key points

- Assessment of menstrual blood loss is highly subjective.
- Some women accept very heavy bleeding as normal.
- Other women can be anxious about a light loss.

Key points (continued)

- Some conditions will cause:
  - irregular bleeding
  - post-coital bleeding
  - post-menopausal bleeding.
- Some abnormal bleeding will be pregnancy related.
- The number of menstrual periods a woman can now expect to have is a phenomenon of the second half of the 20th century.
- Frequent pregnancies combined with lactational amenorrhoea (absence of periods associated with breast-feeding) meant that a woman would experience only 30–40 menstrual periods during her entire life, before the widespread adoption of effective contraception.
- The present average is about 400 menstrual cycles (Coulter 1997).
- Endometrial cancer must always be excluded in women over 40.
- Anaemia should be excluded.
- Menorrhagia can affect both intimate and work relationships.
- Women should not be expected to accept menorrhagia as inevitable.

REFERENCES

Coulter A 1997 Why do women complain of menorrhagia? Gynaecology Forum 2 (1): 9–11

Coulter A, Long A, Kelland J et al 1995 Managing menorrhagia. Quality in Health Care 4 (3): 218–226

Effective Health Care 1995 The management of menorrhagia. August 1995, Number 9, ISSN: 0965–0288

Fraser IS 1997 Medical treatments for menorrhagia. Gynaecology Forum 2 (1): 17–20

O'Brien S, Doyle M 1997 Abnormal vaginal bleeding. In: Luesley D (ed) Common conditions in gynaecology. Chapman & Hall, London, Ch 4

Rees M 1997 Menstrual problems. In: McPherson A, Waller D (eds) Women's health, 4th edn. Oxford University Press, Oxford, Ch 10

Sheldon T 1995 Many unnecessary D&Cs and drugs. Health Summary 12 (10): 4–5

FURTHER READING

Gould G 1995 Menorrhagia: care and treatment. Nursing Standard 9 (32): 36–39

Rees M 1997 Menstrual problems. In: McPherson A, Waller D (eds) Women's health, 4th edn. Oxford University Press, Oxford, Ch 10

RESOURCES

Women's Health Concern (leaflets), PO Box 1629, London SW15 2ZL, UK. Tel.: 020 8780 3916.

OVARIAN CANCER

Ovarian cancer is the most common cause of death from a gynae-cological cancer. About 5000 women will be diagnosed with ovarian cancer in the UK each year. Over 4300 of those women will die from ovarian cancer each year. The overall risk of developing ovarian cancer is approximately 1% (Chamberlain 1995).

Ovarian cancer accounts for 6% of all female cancer deaths (Cancer Research Campaign 1997) There are a number of reasons why the death rate is so high, including:

- the disease may be present for some time before it causes any problems
- it is seldom detected at an early stage.

PROGNOSIS

This depends on the staging of the disease.
Percentage surviving 5 years:

Stage 1 – growth limited to one or both ovaries   78%
Stage 2 – growth limited to pelvis   59%
Stage 3 – growth extending to abdominal cavity   23%
Stage 4 – distant disease   14%
Overall survival rate   <30%.

(Cancer Research Campaign 1997)

SYMPTOMS

There are frequently vague and non-specific symptoms of mild gastrointestinal disturbance, which are often ignored, also:

- abdominal discomfort
- abdominal swelling
- anorexia, weight loss and malaise
- pressure symptoms, particularly affecting bladder and bowel.

RISK FACTORS

Risk factors for developing ovarian cancer:

- Age: 90% of cases occur in women over 45 years (RCN 1995).
- Social class and ethnicity: the disease is more common in white women from higher social class.
- Heredity:
  - 5–10% of ovarian cancers may be hereditary, particularly if it occurs before the age of 50
  - 1 in 40 risk if a woman has a first-degree relative (e.g. mother or sister) diagnosed with the disease before the age of 50
  - 1 in 3 risk if there are two first-degree relatives similarly affected
  - occurs more commonly in families in which other members have breast or bowel cancer.
- Parity:
  - it is more common in women who have not had any children
  - the risk decreases with the number of pregnancies.
- Ovulation:
  - raised risk with a late menopause and a history of infertility
  - there is a possible association with length of years of menstruation (Redman 1997).
- Other factors may include obesity and use of talc in the genital area, but the evidence is inconclusive (Cancer Research Campaign 1997).

SCREENING

Screening for ovarian cancer:

- Blood test measuring serum CA125 (a tumour marker) and vaginal ultrasound, combined with colour Doppler tests (measuring blood flow) should only be offered to women with a family history, because of an otherwise very high false positive rate (Kochli 1995).
- Ultrasound is not reliable in discriminating between benign and malignant tumours: its main role is to identify solid tumours in young women (Chamberlain 1995).
- Bimanual pelvic examination cannot distinguish between malignant and benign tumours and therefore is not acceptable as a screening tool (RCN 1995).

- Bimanual pelvic examination should be used to assess symptomatic women and then only be carried out by those who have been appropriately trained, and who have maintained their skills (RCN 1995).

Nursing issues

Spend some time thinking about the following:

- awareness of the importance of early detection and diagnosis to optimize the prognosis
- knowledge of the impact, on both the woman and her family, of a diagnosis with a poor overall survival rate
- knowledge of some of the treatment and management options
- awareness that for the best prognosis at any stage the initial surgery should be carried out by a specialist skilled in treating ovarian cancer
- awareness of the importance of taking a full family history and the possible need for family genetic counselling
- awareness of issues around screening, including genetic screening
- knowledge of appropriate local and national resources.

DIAGNOSIS

Diagnosis is frequently made late in the disease process:

- <75% of women present with advanced disease: stages 3–4 (Redman 1997)
- ultrasound can demonstrate the presence of a pelvic mass
- surgery is needed for a full assessment of the disease.

TREATMENT

Surgery is the main form of treatment; chemotherapy may be used before or after surgery depending on the extent of the disease and the size of any tumour:

- In Stage I disease the surgery alone can be curative.
- In advanced disease surgery may be used:
  - to reduce or remove all demonstrable disease before chemotherapy
  - to reduce further the size of a large mass (cystoreduction) after chemotherapy has made it more manageable.

Chemotherapy

- The chemotherapy currently in use (platinum-based) extends disease-free survival, but has little impact on the overall cure rate.
- A new group of drugs (taxanes), derived from yew (*Taxus baccata*) have improved results for initial and recurrent disease, and are being further researched (Cancer Research Campaign 1997).

Radiotherapy has little part to play in the adjuvant (add-on) therapy of ovarian cancer.

Key points

- Only rare hormone-secreting tumours affect menstruation.
- The majority of ovarian cancers are epithelial in origin.
  - There is a decreased risk of ovarian cancer:
  - with past oral contraceptive use
  - following sterilization.
- There is not yet any evidence that early detection by screening reduces mortality.
- There are research trials underway to test the usefulness of serum CA125 levels as a predictor of early ovarian cancer in asymptomatic post-menopausal women (Cancer Research Campaign 1997).

REFERENCES

Cancer Research Campaign 1997 Ovarian Cancer – UK. Factsheet 17
Chamberlain G (ed) 1995 Gynaecology by ten teachers, 16th edn. Arnold, London, Ch 6
Kochli OR 1995 Screening women for ovarian cancer: problems and perspectives. Oncology in Practice, July: 90–101
RCN 1995 Bimanual pelvic examination: guidance for nurses. Issues in nursing and health: 34. Royal College of Nursing, London
Redman C 1997 Gynaecological cancers. In: Luesley D (ed) Common conditions in gynaecology. Chapman & Hall, London, Ch 10

FURTHER READING

CancerBACUP Understanding cancer of the ovary. 3 Bath Place, London EC2A 3DR
Gould D 1990 Neoplasms of the female genital tract. In: Gould D, Nursing care of Women. Prentice Hall, Hemel Hempstead, Ch 12

RESOURCE

Cancer Support Service, Information Tel. 020 7613 2121.

OVARIAN CYSTS

Ovarian cysts are usually fluid-filled cysts arising from the ovary, some may be malignant (see p. 307)

SYMPTOMS

There may be no symptoms and the discovery of the cyst may be an incidental finding. Some cysts cause disruption to the menstrual cycle. Some only cause problems when they have grown so large that there is pressure on other organs (e.g. bladder or bowel) or that there is noticeable abdominal swelling. Torsion (twisting) or rupture of a cyst can cause considerable pain.

Torsion:

- may be of the cyst alone if the pedicle is sufficiently long
- may be of the entire ovary.

There are different types of ovarian cysts

TYPES OF CYST
Functional ovarian cysts

Functional ovarian cysts are associated with ovulation.

- Follicular cysts:
  - are common
  - rarely exceed 5 cm in diameter
  - are usually unilateral
  - usually resolve spontaneously.
- Luteal cysts:
  - may disturb menstruation
  - rupture or haemorrhage into the cyst can result in acute lower abdominal pain
  - may be mistaken for an ectopic pregnancy.

Dermoid cysts

Dermoid cysts:

- arise from the germ cell
- are the most common tumour in young women
- are more likely to be associated with torsion
- are solid (may contain teeth, hair, bone, muscle, thyroid and nervous tissue)
- are almost invariably benign
- 20% are bilateral (Chamberlain 1995).

Benign epithelial cysts

Serous and mucinous cystodermas may become very large, leading to abdominal distension. Torsion and haemorrhage can occur.

Endometriotic cysts

These cysts contain blood. When old blood becomes thick and tarry it is termed a 'chocolate' cyst.

Theca lutein cysts

Theca lutein cysts are associated with hydatidiform mole and excessive doses of drugs used to induce ovulation in treatment of infertility (hyperstimulation of the ovaries) (see p. 147).

TREATMENT

Treatment will depend on a definitive diagnosis. Ultrasound scanning is increasingly being used to distinguish between the different types of ovarian cyst and to monitor, as appropriate, therefore reducing the need for surgery.

- Functional cysts:
  - ultrasound scanning can be used to monitor the cyst
  - will usually resolve.
- Torsion of a cyst:
  - will result in considerable pain
  - is a gynaecological emergency
  - if left untreated the cyst will become necrotic
  - laparotomy is essential.

- Rupture of a cyst:
  - if the cyst is large there may be severe pain and shock from bleeding into the peritoneum
  - rupture is most likely to occur with a rapidly growing cyst, that may be malignant (Chamberlain 1995).

Surgery

The extent of the surgery will depend on the type of cyst, the severity of the symptoms, the age of the woman and whether she has started or completed her family.

- Cystectomy, attempting to conserve as much ovarian tissue as possible.
- Oophorectomy (removal of ovary).
- Laparoscopic treatment of torsion has a high recurrence rate (Pickrell 1997).
- Bilateral salpingo-oophorectomy is usually advised in the peri-menopausal or post-menopausal woman (Steele 1997).

Nursing issues

Spend some time thinking about the following:

- knowledge of the incidence and effects of ovarian cysts
- knowledge of monitoring techniques and surgical interventions
- awareness of anxiety and concern about possible malignancy considered by many women
- awareness of issues around future fertility
- awareness of the impact of emergency surgery on any woman and her family.

Key points

- Malignancy must always be excluded.
- The other ovary must be assessed.
- Differential diagnosis, other conditions can have similar signs and symptoms, e.g.
  - ectopic pregnancy
  - fibroids
  - chronic pelvic infection
  - appendicitis or other intestinal disease.
- Polycystic ovarian syndrome (PCOS) (see p. 318) is characterized by:
  - multiple cystic follicles
  - cysts are small
  - increased risk of hyperstimulation in ovulation induction (Pickrell 1997).

REFERENCES

Chamberlain G (ed) 1995 Gynaecology by ten teachers, 16th edn. Arnold, London, Ch 6
Pickrell D 1997 Gynaecological emergencies. In: Luesley D (ed) Common conditions in gynaecology. Chapman & Hall, London, Ch 3
Steele J 1997 Common gynaecological problems. In: Andrews G (ed) Women's sexual health. Baillière Tindall, London, Ch 16

RESOURCE

Women's Health Concern (leaflets and information), PO Box 1629, London SW 15 2ZL, UK. Tel.: 020 8780 3916.

PELVIC INFLAMMATORY DISEASE

Pelvic inflammatory disease (PID) is an infection caused by micro-organisms ascending the genital tract through the cervix. The endometrium, uterine tubes, ovaries, pelvic and abdominal peritoneum can be affected. The infection is usually sexually transmitted and is poorly diagnosed. The organisms most commonly found are *Chlamydia* and *Neisseria gonorrhoeae* or both. Other causative organisms can be *Staphylococcus aureus* and anaerobes. PID has a significant effect on fertility, by damaging the uterine tubes (Oakeshott 1997).

PID may begin with an acute episode that can be completely resolved or which subsides into a chronic condition and it may not be recognized until the damage has been done (Chamberlain 1995).

Less commonly, PID may be caused by surgery (curettage, termination of pregnancy, hysteroscopy, etc.), transperitoneal (appendicitis, abdominal surgery), blood-borne infection (e.g. tuberculosis) (Steele 1997).

Infertility

Infertility following pelvic inflammatory disease is shown in Table 8.3.

Table 8.3   Infertility after PID (Pickrell 1997)

Number of attacks	Percentage infertile
One	11%
Two	23%
Three or more	50%

Nursing issues

Spend some time thinking about the following:

- awareness that the woman can be very ill
- awareness that PID is a major cause of acute admission to hospital
- knowledge of the treatment, including ensuring understanding of the importance of full compliance and follow-up
- understanding of the importance of contact tracing
- understanding the importance of dealing sensitively with all issues around sexual health
- knowledge of the devastating effect that PID can have on fertility
- awareness of the long-term effects, physical and psychological, of chronic PID.

Incidence

PID is (Church & Sutton 1996):

- never found before puberty
- rare after the menopause
- only found in sexually active women
- most commonly found in young women aged between 15 and 24 years.

Symptoms

Common symptoms are:

- lower abdominal pain
- pyrexia, headache, malaise
- vaginal discharge
- dyspareunia
- irregular vaginal bleeding.

Signs of PID

Examination demonstrates:

- bimanual tenderness
- pyrexia
- cervical motion tenderness (cervical excitation)
- bimanual mass
- purulent vaginal discharge.

Predisposing factors

These are (Chamberlain 1995):

- current IUD use (possibly by reactivating pre-existing infection)
- history of previous attacks
- history of previous STI
- partner has STI.

Differential diagnosis

PID may be confused with:

- appendicitis
- endometriosis
- ectopic pregnancy.

Diagnosis

PID is not always easily diagnosed. There are diagnostic criteria (Church & Sutton 1996):

- Diagnosis is presumed if there are the following findings:
  - abdominal tenderness on examination
  - cervical excitation
  - adnexal tenderness on examination (ovaries and uterine tubes)
  - pyrexia
  - raised white cell count.
- Urethral, vaginal and cervical swabs must be taken and tested for *Chlamydia* and gonorrhoea.
- Pelvic ultrasound (see p. 344) may demonstrate an abcess
- Laparoscopy may be indicated where there is doubt about the diagnosis.

TREATMENT

Treatment is (Adler 1995):

- bedrest
- removal of IUD (if present) once treatment has started
- antibiotic treatment should be started before microbiological results are known
- non-gonococccal infection – metronidazole plus tetracycline or doxycycline for 10–14 days
- gonococcal infection – penicillin or amoxycillin
- abstaining from sexual intercourse
- tracing and treating partners (if *Chlamydia* or gonorrhoea suspected or diagnosed).

Consequences of PID

These can be:

- chronic pelvic pain
- menstrual disturbances
- dyspareunia
- infertility
- ectopic pregnancy
- relationship difficulties (because of the pain or the possible betrayal of trust).

Key point
Some women are so affected by their PID that they consider hysterectomy.

REFERENCES

Adler M (ed) 1995 ABC of sexually transmitted diseases. BMJ, London
Chamberlain G (ed) 1995 Gynaecology by ten teachers, 16th edn. Arnold, London, Ch 5
Church N, Sutton A 1996 Chlamydia and pelvic inflammatory disease. In: Sutton A, Payne S (eds) Genito-urinary medicine for nurses. Whurr, London, Ch 6
Oakeshott P 1997 Vaginal discharge and sexually transmitted diseases. In: McPherson A, Waller D (eds) Women's health, 4th edn. Oxford University Press, Oxford, Ch 13
Pickrell D 1997 Gynaecological emergencies. In: Luesley D (ed) Common conditions in gynaecology. Chapman & Hall, London, Ch 3

Steele J 1997 Common gynaecological problems. In: Andrews G (ed) Women's sexual health. Baillière Tindall, London, Ch 16

RESOURCE

Health Education Authority (leaflet), 30 Great Peter Street, London SW 1 8RT, UK. Tel.: 020 7222 5300

POLYCYSTIC OVARY SYNDROME

Polycystic ovary syndrome (PCOS) is a common endocrine disorder in which there are the following elements:

- an excessive number of small, cystic follicles around the ovary
- failure of ovulation
- a continuous background of oestrogen production by the small follicles (non-cyclical)
- thickened ovarian stroma producing excessive androgens
- disrupted follicle stimulating hormone/luteinizing hormone (FSH/LH) ratio.

INCIDENCE AND SYMPTOMS

PCOS is present in:

- 90% of women with oligomenorrhoea
- 30% of women with amenorrhoea
- 20% of 'normal' population with irregular periods
- 7% of women with regular periods (Rees 1993).

Classically, this condition is characterized as:

- amenorrhoea
- hirsutism
- obesity
- bilateral polycystic ovaries.

However, there can be any type of menstrual irregularity: e.g. oligomenorrhoea, irregular/infrequent periods or menorrhagia.

Other signs are those of hyperandrogenism, caused by raised levels of serum testosterone such as:

- acne
- androgenic alopecia (male-pattern baldness).

PCOS AND INFERTILITY

PCOS is also associated with infertility, which could be caused by:

- anovulation
- high circulating levels of LH (probably inhibiting ovum development within the follicle, and embryo implantation within the uterus, should the woman conceive).

PCOS accounts for 73% of anovulatory infertility (Hull et al 1985).

DIAGNOSIS

Diagnosis is by:

- history and observation
- transvaginal pelvic ultrasound to confirm the presence of polycystic ovaries (the multiple cystic follicles being described as 'a string of pearls') (see p. 344)
- exclusion of other disorders of hypothalamic–pituitary–ovarian axis (see p. 96)
- hormonal tests, testing for levels of:
  - LH
  - FSH
  - testosterone
  - prolactin
  - sex hormone binding globulin.

These tests may be of some value in confirming a diagnosis.

TREATMENT

This is usually symptomatic, but may include ovulation induction if a pregnancy is wanted. For the woman who wants to become pregnant drugs will be needed to induce ovulation (see p. 146).

There are two types of ovulation induction:

1. Clomiphene citrate (an anti-oestrogen, which stimulates endogenous FSH production) for up to six cycles:
   - women with abnormally high serum LH levels (over 10 iu/l) have reduced chance of success and a higher rate of miscarriage
   - ovulation induced in over 80% of women
   - 40% pregnancy rate

- clomiphene therapy should not be given for more than 6 months because of the perceived risk of ovarian cancer (Balen 1995):
2. Gonadotrophin therapy is indicated in women who have been treated with anti-oestrogens and:
   - have failed to ovulate
   - have persistent hypersecretion of LH
   - have had a negative post-coital test (due to the effect of anti-oestrogens on cervical mucus)
   - additional pituitary control with LHRH analogues, to suppress LH production may be necessary.

Gonadotrophin therapy:

- Carries risks and should be carried out in a specialist unit with appropriate monitoring.
- Is associated with a higher incidence of multiple pregnancies (19%).
- Carries a risk of ovarian hyperstimulation (see p. 147).
- There is a possible association between induced multiple ovulations or superovulation therapies and ovarian cancer.

Surgical treatment

Laparoscopic ovarian diathermy has replaced ovarian wedge resection for the management of clomiphene resistance in women with PCOS (Balen 1995). The advantages include:

- no increased risk of multiple pregnancies
- no risk of ovarian hyperstimulation
- not requiring intensive ultrasound monitoring
- diathermy to one ovary leads to bilateral ovarian activity.

The disadvantages include:

- difficulty of access to appropriately trained laparoscopic surgeon
- uncertainty about minimum dose of diathermy needed.

Treatment for the woman who does not want to become pregnant, is at present:

- Cyproterone acetate (Dianette) which reduces testosterone levels, so helping greasy skin, acne and excess body hair; it also produces a regular withdrawal bleed, and also provides contraception.

- A 30 µg contraceptive pill (e.g. Microgynon or Ovranette) may reduce some less severe symptoms, as well as providing a withdrawal bleed and contraception.
- Non-androgenic progestagens (e.g. medroxyprogesterone acetate, desogestrel and gestodene) given cyclically produce a regular withdrawal bleed.

Nursing issues

Spend some time thinking about the following:

- knowledge of the incidence and spectrum of characteristics of PCOS
- awareness of concerns around fertility
- understand that the physical signs of severe disease can be very distressing and may prevent a woman from taking part in a full life and forming intimate relationships
- understanding that minimal overt physical symptoms may not reflect the extent of the problem
- supporting weight reduction in obese women with PCOS is key to their care:
  - many have an abnormal lipid profile
  - many are at increased risk of atherosclerosis and cardiovascular disease in later life
  - loss of more than 5% of initial body weight results in marked improvement in clinical and endocrine function and possible return of ovulation (Kiddy et al 1995)
  - weight loss, combined with increased fitness through exercise, and psychological support to improve self-esteem can significantly improve pregnancy and ovulation rates (Clark et al 1995)
- awareness that nurses should:
  - be able to describe treatment options
  - have a knowledge of drugs used
  - be aware of available resources
  - note that some women gain benefits from alternative therapies, such as zinc, agnus castus and aloe-vera; however there is only anecdotal evidence to support these claims.

Key points

- Not every woman with PCOS will be hirsute or have other signs of hyperandrogenism.
- Obese women (BMI greater than 30) are found to hypersecrete insulin, which stimulates the ovaries to secrete androgens.
- Obese women with PCOS are at greatly increased risk of developing non-insulin diabetes mellitus (NIDDM).
- Increased exposure to oestrogens predisposes to endometrial hyperplasia, which can be a precursor for endometrial cancer:
  - obese women have higher levels of oestrogens resulting from more androstenedione being converted to oestrone by adipose tissue
  - high levels of oestrogen in women who have anovulatory cycles (Redman 1997).

REFERENCES

Balen A 1995 Ovulation disorders and polycystic ovary syndrome. Update Postgraduate Centre Series: Infertility, Reed Healthcare Communications

Clark AM, Ledger W, Galletly C, Tomlinson L, Blaney F, Wang X, Norman RJ 1995 Weight loss results in significant improvement in pregnancy and ovulation rates in anovulatory obese women. Human Reproduction 10(10): 2705–2712

Hull MGR, Glazener CM, Kelly MJ 1985 Population study of causes, treatment and outcome of fertility. British Medical Journal 291: 1693–1697

Kiddy D, Corrigan L, Cant S 1995 The nurse's role in specific treatments. In: Meerabeau L, Denton J (eds) Infertility – nursing and caring. Scutari Press, London, Ch 6

Redman C 1997 Gynecological cancers. In: Luesley D (ed) Common conditions in gynaecology. Chapman & Hall Medical, London, Ch 10

Rees M 1993 Menstrual problems. In: McPherson A (ed) Women's problems in general practice, 3rd edn. Oxford University Press, Oxford, Ch 6

RESOURCE

VERITY (self-help group), 30 Chalton House, Chalton Street, London NW1 1HH, UK. Tel.: 020 7388 2949.

VAGINAL DISCHARGE

Vaginal discharge is characterized by secretions from the vagina that can have physiological or pathological causes.

PHYSIOLOGICAL VAGINAL DISCHARGE

This is the normal vaginal discharge, and is made up of secretions from:

- the endocervix
- Bartholin's (vestibular) glands
- Skene's (paraurethral) glands.

It also contains epithelium shed from the vagina and lactobacilli.

Normal vaginal acidity is pH 4.5, an environment in which most pathogens cannot survive. The discharge is clear or whitish in colour, becoming yellow on contact with air due to oxidation, and should not cause soreness, irritation or have an offensive odour.

The quantity varies considerably from woman to woman. There are 'normal' causes for an increase in discharge (Nash 1997):

- cyclically just before ovulation (egg-white appearance)
- premenstrually
- during pregnancy (leucorrhoea)
- contraception (oral contraceptive pill or intrauterine device)
- sexual arousal
- stress.

PATHOLOGICAL VAGINAL DISCHARGE
Infective causes

Common causes include:

- bacterial vaginosis
- *Candida albicans* (thrush)
- *Trichomonas vaginalis*
- *Chlamydia*
- gonorrhoea
- cervical lesions from herpes, warts or syphilis
- streptococcus and staphylococcus.

Non-infective causes

Common causes include:

- cervical ectropion
- cervical polyp
- cervical cancer
- retained products of conception (post-abortion, postnatal)
- 'lost' tampon or condom
- irritants (rubber, latex, spermicide, etc.).

WHAT TO ASK ABOUT THE DISCHARGE

- How is it different from normal?
- Why is she worried about it?
- Are there any other associated symptoms (dysuria, soreness, intermenstrual bleeding, pelvic discomfort)?
- Has anything happened to make her vagina less acidic (is she overwashing with strong soaps using disinfectant in the bath, douching, is she menopausal)?
- Does it have a characteristic smell?

- Does she have any reason to be worried about an STI:
  - change of partner
  - multiple partners
  - partner with urethritis?
- Has she already treated herself unsuccessfully with an over-the-counter (OTC) preparation?

DIAGNOSIS

Diagnosis is by:

- sensitive and thorough history
- assessment of possible risk of STI
- microbiological tests.

Nursing issues

Spend some time thinking about the following:

- knowledge of the normal physiology of the vagina and vaginal secretions
- awareness of the difficulty and embarrassment that many women have in discussing intimate concerns
- awareness of the sensitivity needed to discuss sexual health issues
- knowledge of some cultural and religious practices in relation to personal hygiene
- awareness of the importance of always demonstrating respect and maintaining confidentiality.

Key point

A woman's description of her symptoms and of her discharge 'are a poor guide to the exact nature of the condition' (Adler 1995).

REFERENCES

Adler M (ed) 1995 ABC of sexually transmitted disease, 3rd edn. BMJ, London
Nash J 1997 Sexual health and sexually acquired infection. In: Andrews G (ed) Women's sexual health. Baillière Tindall, London, Ch 12

FURTHER READING

Oakeshott P 1997 Vaginal discharge and sexually transmitted diseases. In: McPherson A, Waller D (eds) Women's health, 4th edn. Oxford University Press, Oxford, Ch 13

9

Some common treatments, procedures and investigations

BREAST SURGERY

There are different types of breast surgery.

SURGERY FOR BREAST CANCER

The type of surgery will depend on a number of factors, including the size, type and spread of the tumour, the age and health of the woman, and her wishes.

Lumpectomy

This is removal of the breast lump and some surrounding tissue, by wide local excision. There is usually a good cosmetic result. Axillary nodes may be sampled at the same time. The breast is conserved.

Quadrantectomy

This is the more extensive excision of a whole quadrant of the breast. Results can look good, except in the woman with small breasts, when it is likely to be more noticeable. Axillary nodes may be sampled. The breast is conserved.

Mastectomy

Removal of the whole breast:

- Simple mastectomy:
  - removal of the whole breast
  - axillary lymph nodes may be sampled.
- Modified radical mastectomy:
  - removal of the whole breast
  - plus the pectoralis minor muscle
  - plus clearance of axillary lymph nodes.
- Radical mastectomy:
  - removal of the whole breast
  - plus the pectoralis major and minor muscles
  - plus clearance of axillary lymph nodes.

BREAST RECONSTRUCTION

A woman may opt for breast reconstruction following surgery for breast cancer. The purpose of the operation is to reconstruct a breast mound to produce breast symmetry (Watson et al 1995).

Reconstruction may be carried out at the time of the original breast surgery or may be deferred until much later. Reconstruction can be:

- immediate replacement with a prosthesis (implant)
- insertion of a tissue expander
- insertion of a flap of skin and muscle (myocutaneous flap) with or without a prosthesis (Watson et al 1995).

OTHER BREAST SURGERY

Breast augmentation (mammoplasty)

A procedure to enlarge the breasts, in which the prosthesis is placed behind the pectoralis major. It is a relatively common procedure for the woman who is dissatisfied with the size of her breasts (she will have to pay for the operation). The procedure can be performed on the woman who has a congenital absence of one breast or one breast considerably smaller than the other.

Breast reduction

Breast reduction is a procedure involving the removal of breast tissue, and is considered a cosmetic procedure for the woman

---

Nursing issues

Spend some time thinking about the following:
- knowledge of different types of breast surgery
- understanding that women with breast cancer are actively involved in making decisions about their treatment
- awareness of the role of and means of referral to the specialist breast care nurse, who has a significant role in supporting women with breast cancer and their families; before, during and after diagnosis and treatment
- awareness of the impact of any breast surgery on a woman's body image and sexuality
- awareness of the impact of breast surgery on a woman's partner
- knowledge of local and national support groups and resources.

Key points

- Extent of local surgery does not appear to influence survival.
- Breast conservation surgery should be supplemented by radiotherapy.
- Radical mastectomy should rarely be carried out, since studies comparing radical mastectomy with quadrantectomy have shown overall survival, and survival without relapse, were identical with the two treatments.
- Other studies have shown that lumpectomies followed by whole breast radiotherapy provide similar rates of local control and survival to that seen with quadrantectomy or simple mastectomy. (Riley & Baum 1995).
- Myocutaneous flap reconstructions will leave scars on areas other than the breast (e.g. on the back).
- Fibrous capsules can develop around prostheses.
- All forms of breast reconstruction are substantial surgical operations that should be carried out by experienced surgeons.
- Some women may have unrealistic expectations of how augmentation will change their body image, personality or lifestyle (Edge & Miller 1994).

who is dissatisfied with the size of her breasts. The procedure may be recommended for the woman whose breasts (or just one breast) are so large that they cause physical or psychological problems or interfere with her life and physical activities.

REFERENCES

Edge V, Miller M (eds) 1994 Therapeutic and elective procedures and surgeries. In: Women's health care. Mosby, St. Louis
Riley D, Baum M 1995 Clinical trials of management of breast cancer. In: Dixon JM (ed) ABC of breast diseases. BMJ Publishing, London
Watson JD, Sainsbury JRC, Dixon JM 1995 Breast reconstruction. In: Dixon JM (ed) ABC of breast diseases. BMJ Publishing, London

FURTHER READING

Curling G, Tierney K 1997 Breast screening and breast disorders. In: Andrews G (ed) Women's sexual health. Baillière Tindall, London
Denton S 1996 Breast cancer nursing. Chapman & Hall, London
Edge V, Miller M (eds) 1994 Therapeutic and elective procedures and surgeries. In: Women's health care. Mosby, St. Louis

RESOURCES

Breast Cancer Care, Kiln House, 210 New Kings Road, London SW6 4NZ, UK. Administration: 020 7384 2984; Helpline: 020 7384 2344; Nationwide freeline: 0500 245 345.
CancerBACUP, 3 Bath Place, Rivington Street, London EC2A 3DR, UK. Cancer Support Service, Information: 020 7613 2121; Freeline: 0800 18 11 99.

COLPOSCOPY

Colposcopy is a procedure carried out using a colposcope (Fig. 9.1), which is a binocular microscope designed to magnify the cervix under a bright light. It can also be used to examine the vagina, vulva and anus. The purpose of the examination is to visualize the transformation zone at the squamocolumnar junction. It is used for the following reasons:

- metaplasia occurs within the transformation zone where the original columnar cells are replaced by columnar epithelium
- abnormal metaplasia, or dysplasia, is known as cervical intraepithelial neoplasia (CIN) and is considered a pre-cancerous condition

- every woman with an abnormal cervical smear suggesting CIN should have a colposcopic examination.

During the procedure a further smear may be taken, a biopsy performed and some treatments carried out (see p. 340).

Colposcopy is usually carried out in out-patient gynaecology clinics or in dedicated colposcopy clinics. A few GPs have facilities in their own practices. Wherever colposcopy is carried out there should be strict adherence to following the guidelines and achieving the *Standards & Quality in Colposcopy* as set out by the NHSCSP.

There are referral criteria for colposcopy, which are usually dependent on a women's smear result:

- borderline smear on two or three occasions
- mild dyskaryosis (abnormal nucleus) on two occasions
- moderate dyskaryosis on one occasion
- severe dyskaryosis on one occasion
- inadequate smear on three occasions
- any woman with a clinically suspicious cervix, regardless of her smear result.

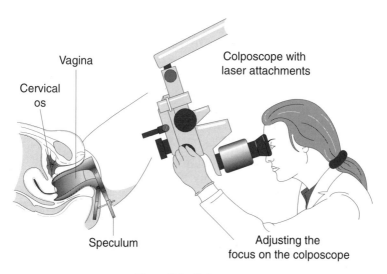

Figure 9.1   Colposcopy

Nursing issues

Spend some time thinking about the following:

- understanding that privacy must be maintained at all times
- awareness that this is the most lengthy and intimate procedure that most women will experience
- the procedure cannot be carried out if the woman is menstruating
- ability to explain exactly what is going to happen
- ability to provide information, comfort and support, preserving the woman's dignity at all times
- some nurses have undertaken specialist training and can perform the procedure, so providing total patient care
- awareness that although this is supposed to be a virtually painless procedure, some women find it extremely painful/traumatic
- understanding that this is one of the consequences of screening healthy women (if you screen enough women sufficiently rigorously you are bound to find something)
- making sure the woman understands how to care for herself after the procedure, including when to seek medical advice
- information about any discharge/bleeding following the procedure (how much and for how long)
- ensuring an understanding of any follow-up consultations
- colposcopy units should send out a detailed information leaflet prior to the appointment.

What any woman should have explained to her about colposcopy:

- she will be told of any procedure before it happens
- she lies on a couch/chair with her legs in rests
- the colposcope does not enter her vagina, only a speculum does
- the procedure usually takes 10–15 minutes
- she is informed of the diagnosis and treatment options discussed
- she consents to any further treatment
- adequate pain relief is available
- she will be given written information to take away
- she cannot necessarily insist on a female doctor.

When a woman is referred for colposcopy she should be prepared for (Austoker & Davey 1997):

- the procedure of colposcopy
- possible embarrassment due to the lithotomy position
- the possibility of a cervical biopsy
- the possibility that treatment may occur with the initial examination
- likely treatment options.

The procedure:

- the woman is in the lithotomy position
- a Cusco speculum is used to expose the cervix
- dilute acetic acid is painted onto the cervix, temporarily staining abnormal epithelium white
- sometimes an iodine solution is used (normal epithelium will stain dark brown), but is considered less discriminatory as to the nature, merely indicating the extent of the area (Chamberlain 1995)
- the transformation zone (TZ) must be examined, this may be difficult in older women when it may be out of view up the endocervical canal
- biopsies are taken from the abnormal areas, to confirm the diagnosis and exclude the possibility of invasive disease
- if the TZ is seen and histology confirms pre-invasive disease then conservative treatment can be carried out
- some treatments may be carried out straightaway for minor abnormalities (see p. 340).

REFERENCES

Austoker J, Davey C 1997 Cervical smear results explained: a guide for primary care. Cancer Research Campaign, London
Chamberlain G (ed) 1995 Gynaecological tumours. In: Gynaecology by ten teachers, 16th edn. Arnold, London, Ch 6
National Health Service Cervical Screening Programme 1996 Publication No 2 Luesley D (ed) Standards & quality in colposcopy

GYNAECOLOGICAL SURGERY AND INVESTIGATIONS

There are a number of commonly performed gynaecological procedures and investigations.

DILATATION AND CURETTAGE (D&C)

D&C is the commonest minor gynaecological procedure in which the endometrium is sampled or removed. It may be used as a *diagnostic* test to determine the cause of heavy, long or irregular periods, intermenstrual bleeding, post-coital bleeding or post-menopausal bleeding. It may be performed as a *therapeutic* procedure (e.g. to remove an endometrial polyp, or after an incomplete abortion).

D&C does not sample the whole of the endometrium (Rees 1997). It is usually carried out under general anaesthetic.

Diagnostic D&C should not be performed on women aged under 40, since it is an unnecessary procedure, and its use could be replaced by cheaper and safer methods of endometrial sampling (see later) (Effective Health Care 1995).

Risks of D&C include possible perforation of the uterus and damage to the cervix through over-dilatation.

ENDOMETRIAL BIOPSY (BY ASPIRATION CURETTAGE)

This is a diagnostic test to determine the cause of heavy, long or irregular periods, intermenstrual bleeding, post-coital bleeding or post-menopausal bleeding.

During the procedure a fine tube is passed through the cervix into the uterine cavity and a sample of endometrium is sucked out.

The procedure is usually carried out in an outpatient clinic, and can be carried out with either no anaesthetic or local anaesthetic, carrying fewer risks than D&C. The woman should feel little pain or discomfort when the procedure is carried out skillfuly.

HYSTERECTOMY

This is the surgical removal of the uterus.

There are different types of hysterectomy:

- total: the uterus and cervix are removed
- subtotal: the uterus alone is removed
- radical: the uterus, cervix, the upper third of the vagina, pelvic lymph nodes, uterine tubes and ovaries are removed.

The type of hysterectomy will depend on the reason for the operation.

Reasons for hysterectomy include:

- cancer in the genital tract
- heavy periods or dysfunctional uterine bleeding
- fibroids
- uterine prolapse

- chronic pelvic infection
- severe endometriosis (see p. 287).

A vaginal hysterectomy is usually carried out for uterine prolapse (see p. 298).

In the absence of malignancy or if the woman is under 50 years old the ovaries are usually left, but they are frequently removed, despite being healthy, to prevent a theoretical risk of developing ovarian cancer.

If a subtotal hysterectomy is carried out, the woman should continue having routine cervical smears. If a hysterectomy is carried out for a malignant or premalignant condition of the cervix, annual vault smears should be performed for at least two or three years.

Key points

- The woman who has conserved her ovaries at the time of hysterectomy is still more likely to experience an earlier menopause, probably because of compromise to the blood supply to the ovaries.
- For non-malignant conditions the wishes of the woman are paramount.

OTHER OPERATIONS

Hysterosalpingogram

This procedure is commonly carried out as part of investigation for infertility and is X-ray imaging of the uterine cavity and uterine tubes to demonstrate abnormality of the uterine cavity and patency of the tubes. During the procedure a radio-opaque dye is injected into the uterus via the cervix and if the tubes are patent the dye passes into the peritoneal cavity.

It is important prior to planned tubal surgery to define the level and extent of tubal damage. The procedure is now more likely to be reserved for the woman for whom laparoscopy is contraindicated (Blunt & Walker 1997).

Hysteroscopy

In this procedure a small fibre-optic telescope is passed through the cervix so that the uterine cavity and endometrium can be visualized. It may identify endometrial polyps or fibroids. It can be carried out in outpatient clinics and a local anaesthetic should be used. The procedure is best reserved for women with persistent bleeding where endometrial biopsy is negative or the endometrium is found to be abnormally thickened on ultrasound (Rees 1997).

Procedures for infertility

There are a number of surgical procedures that may be carried out to improve fertility, e.g.:

- reversal of sterilization, when a woman wants another baby after being sterilized, possibly with a new partner
- tubal microsurgery, for uterine tubes that have been damaged by infection
- diathermy or laser to endometriotic deposits, particularly those on the surface of the ovary
- surgery or laser to the ovary for polycystic ovary syndrome (PCOS) (see p. 318) may improve ovulation
- correction of uterine abnormalities (e.g. septum in uterus and vagina caused by mid-line fusion problems during fetal development).

Myomectomy

This is the removal of a fibroid and is usually performed by an open operative procedure, but submucous fibroids may be removed via a hysteroscope (O'Brien & Doyle 1997). The fibroid may recur, therefore hysterectomy is usually advised for the woman whose fibroids are a problem.

Myomectomy is likely to be reserved for the woman who has not started or completed her family.

Salpingectomy

This is the surgical removal of the uterine tube and may be carried out for ectopic pregnancy or chronic tubal infection.

Oophorectomy

This is the surgical removal of the ovary, usually for cancer, cysts or possibly endometriosis. Ovarian cystectomy is the surgical removal of a benign ovarian cyst.

Ovarian wedge resection is the removal of about one-third of the ovary, and is a procedure that may be carried out for PCOS.

'Repair' operations

These are surgical procedures to repair or correct genital prolapse and/or urinary incontinence (see p. 268) and may be carried out via vaginal or abdominal route depending on the woman's symptoms and the surgeon's skills and preference.

Procedures include:

Anterior colporrhaphy

This is the repair of the anterior vaginal wall and is performed vaginally. The procedure is indicated for cystocele and cystourethrocele, with or without stress incontinence. However, it may be a less effective cure for incontinence than suprapubic operations (Chamberlain 1995).

Posterior colporrhaphy

This is the repair of the posterior vaginal wall and is performed vaginally. The procedure is indicated for rectocele, or rectocele and enterocele.

Surgery for stress incontinence

Colposuspension may be indicated in which a variety of procedures are used to elevate the bladder neck. Artificial sphincters, slings and injectables (e.g. collagen) can improve urinary control. Sphincter repair or reconstruction may be the appropriate treatment.

Vaginal hysterectomy

This may may be used for moderate/severe uterine prolapse. However, it can only be carried out if the uterus is smaller than the size of a 14-week pregnancy and there is no genital tract malignancy.

Vaginal vault suspension

This procedure is used to repair a prolapse of the vaginal vault, which can occur following hysterectomy.

Transcervical resection of the endometrium (TCRE)

This is the surgical removal of the endometrium through the cervix whilst conserving the uterus (O'Brien & Doyle 1997) and is also called endometrial ablation. The procedure is considered by some to be an alternative to hysterectomy and is used in the management of menorrhagia (see p. 302). However, not all women with menorrhagia will be suitable for the procedure.

Vulvectomy

This is the surgical removal of the vulva and may be one of two procedures. Simple vulvectomy is the removal of the labia and possibly the clitoris and is carried out for vulval intraepithelial neoplasia (VIN), vulval dystrophy or intractable pruritus vulvae. Radical vulvectomy is the extensive removal of the vulval tissue and inguinal lymph nodes, and is carried out for cancer of the vulva (Chamberlain 1995).

More than any other gynaecological surgery, vulvectomy and radical vulvectomy have a huge effect on a woman's self-esteem, body image and sexuality, and wide-ranging implications for the woman, her partner and family (Rider 1997).

Nursing issues

Spend some time thinking about the following:

- knowledge of the surgical procedures used for gynaecological disorder and disease
- knowledge of specific procedures most commonly carried out by specialists in own region and any preparation necessary for that procedure
- understanding the need for the woman to choose the type and extent of surgery, as far as possible
- understanding the need to communicate clearly all issues around convalescence and recovery
- awareness of the impact of gynaecological surgery on body image and sexual functioning; for some there may be fear that a gynaecological cancer can be sexually transmitted, while for others it may be necessary to discuss different positions and means to achieve sexual satisfaction
- awareness of the effect on the woman's partner, family and other relationships
- awareness of the distress of fertility issues
- understanding and demonstrating respect for individual social, cultural and religious beliefs
- knowledge of local and national resources, self-help groups and information.

REFERENCES

Blunt S, Walker D 1997 Infertility and pregnancy loss. In: Luesley D (ed) Common conditions in gynaecology. Chapman & Hall, London, Ch 7

Chamberlain G (ed) 1995 Therapy. In: Gynaecology by ten teachers, 16th edn. Arnold, London, Ch 13

Effective Health Care 1995 The management of menorrhagia. NHS Centre for Reviews and Dissemination, York

O'Brien S, Doyle M 1997 Abnormal vaginal bleeding. In: Luesley D (ed) Common conditions in gynaecology. Chapman & Hall, London, Ch 4

Rees M 1997 Menstrual problems. In: McPherson A, Waller D (eds) Women's health, 4th edn. Oxford University Press, Oxford, Ch 10

Rider I 1997 Gynaecological investigations and surgery. In: Andrews G (ed) Women's sexual health. Baillière Tindall, London, Ch 17

FURTHER READING

Gould D 1990 Nursing care of women. Prentice Hall, New York

Haslett S, Jennings M 1998 Hysterectomy and vaginal repair, 4th edn. Beaconsfield Publishers, Beaconsfield

National Osteoporosis Society and the RCN Gynaecological Nursing Forum 1996 Hysterectomy advice pack. National Osteoporosis Society, Bath

Rider I 1997 Gynaecological investigations and surgery. In: Andrews G (ed) Women's sexual health. Baillière Tindall, London

RESOURCES

CancerBACUP, 3 Bath Place, Rivington Street, London EC2A 3JR, UK. Cancer Information Service, 020 7613 2121, Freeline 0800 18 11 99.

Hysterectomy Support Network, 210 Heath Road, Lawrence Cottages, Orett Heath, Grays, Essex RM16 3AP, UK.

Women's Health Concern, PO Box 1629, London SW15 2ZL, UK. Tel.: 020 8780 3916.

LAPAROSCOPY

Laparoscopy is a method of visualizing the abdominal and pelvic organs and is a procedure used for diagnosis and for surgical treatment. Visualization is with a fibre-optic light and telescope (laparoscope).

THE PROCEDURE

It is usually carried out under a general anaesthetic, during which a needle is inserted through a small incision in the abdomen (usually just below the umbilicus) and the peritoneal cavity is filled with carbon dioxide gas (2–3 litres) to allow the organs to be viewed easily. The laparoscope is then inserted into the peritoneal cavity. If any procedure is to be carried out a second instrument can be inserted via a further incision, usually in the suprapubic area. At the end of the procedure most of the carbon dioxide is expelled by manual abdominal pressure (Chamberlain 1995).

The woman can usually go home several hours after the procedure, but that will depend on the reason for the laparoscopy.

Carbon dioxide remaining in the peritoneal cavity can result in pain in the abdomen and shoulder for a day or so.

INDICATIONS (Chamberlain 1995)

For diagnosis, e.g.:

- unexplained pelvic pain
- presence and extent of endometriosis
- ovarian tumours and cysts
- adhesions
- tubal infection or ectopic pregnancy
- infertility investigations ('lap and dye' is the procedure in which dye is introduced into the uterus via the cervix to see if it then spills out into the peritoneal cavity).

For therapeutic use, e.g.:

- sterilization
- division of adhesions
- puncture of benign ovarian cysts
- hysterectomy
- laser ablation of endometriotic deposits
- ectopic pregnancy
- tubal surgery.

Nursing issues

Spend some time thinking about the following:

- knowledge of the procedure and any preparation that may be necessary
- knowledge of whether laparoscopy is being carried out for diagnostic or therapeutic reasons
- awareness of issues around fertility, infertility and sexuality
- awareness of the distress of the woman with an ectopic pregnancy.

REFERENCE

Chamberlain G (ed) 1995 Therapy. In: Gynaecology by ten teachers, 16th edn. Arnold, London, Ch 13

FURTHER READING

Rider I 1997 Gynaecological investigations and surgery. In: Andrews G (ed) Women's sexual health. Baillière Tindall, London, Ch 17

CERVICAL INTRAEPITHELIAL NEOPLASIA (CIN)

There are principles for the treatment of CIN:

- conservative treatment is used whenever possible, especially in younger women who may not have started or completed their family.
- approximately 70% of women with smears and biopsies showing CIN 3 can be treated conservatively, so avoiding cone biopsy (Chamberlain 1995).

There are treatment standards in colposcopy set by the National Health Service Cervical Screening Programme (NHSCSP 1996) covering such issues as:

- skills level for those who carry out colposcopy and the treatments
- information and communication
- treatment protocols
- anaesthesia
- staffing and equipment
- audit and liaison
- follow-up
- training standards.

METHODS OF TREATMENT

Local destructive therapy:

- carbon dioxide laser ablation
- 'cold' coagulation
- cryosurgery
- electrocoagulation.

Nursing issues

Spend some time thinking about the following:

- recognize the anxiety, fear and even terror that women can have in anticipation of the investigation and treatment
- try to reduce the anxiety by treating each woman as an individual, finding out her particular situation and providing appropriate information for her e.g.:
  - fear of cancer
  - embarrassment at the procedure
  - fear of pain
  - concerns for future fertility
  - worries about further treatment
  - concerns about effects on sexuality
  - belief that CIN is 'dirty' and caused by 'bad' sexual behaviour
- treatment for CIN can have a profound effect on a woman's sexual feelings and behaviour
- support her through the treatment
- ensure that adequate pain relief is available
- ensure she takes away written information on self-care after the treatment (Box 9.1) and advice on when to seek medical attention in the event of difficulties e.g.
  - for how long and what type of discharge she might expect
  - how soon she can resume a sexual relationship
  - tampon use
- a primary nurse working in this setting should be appropriately trained, including having counselling skills
- some nurses have been trained as colposcopists
- reassessment must be made at any stage if any recurrence is suspected.

Local excision:

- large loop excision of the transformation zone (LLETZ)
- knife cone biopsy
- laser cone biopsy.

Carbon dioxide laser ablation

- Laser is the acronym for light amplification by stimulated emission of radiation.
- Waves of infrared light are controlled by the discharge of carbon dioxide.
- The laser destroys the cells by vaporization.
- The beam is very fine and can be sharply directed for both area and depth of destruction.

- There is minimal bleeding.
- The smell of the tissue fumes can be very off-putting.
- Does not effect cervical function.

'Cold' coagulation

- Not cold, but at a lower temperature than laser and loop.
- Tissue is destroyed by the application of heated probes.
- Takes longer than laser to carry out treatment, can be painful.
- Does not affect cervical function.

Cryosurgery

- Tissue is destroyed by the application of freezing probes, usually using nitrous oxide.
- Can be useful for small lesions.
- Large lesions will need multiple applications.
- Depth of tissue destruction difficult to gauge.
- Discharge can be troublesome following treatment.
- Does not affect cervical function.

Electrocoagulation (diathermy)

- Often carried out under general anaesthetic.
- Has largely been superseded by other methods.
- Discharge can be troublesome following treatment.
- Does not affect cervical function.

LLETZ

- Produces a specimen for histological examination.
- Can reduce the need for a biopsy.
- The whole of the transformation zone can be excised.
- Clinics can operate a 'see and treat' policy (Smith 1997).
- There are different sized loops for precision.
- Is considered by many as the routine management of CIN.
- Is generally quick and safe.
- There may be over-treatment of minor abnormalities.
- Has significantly reduced the need for cone biopsy.
- Does not affect cervical function.

Cone Biopsy

Cone biopsy involves the excision of a cone of tissue that should include the whole transformation zone and up to two-thirds of the cervical canal.

Indications for cone biopsy:

- upper limit of lesion cannot be visualized
- microinvasion detected or suspected
- unsuccessful local destructive therapy (persisting or recurring CIN)
- possibly where there has been wide divergence between the cytology and histology reports.

The procedure can be performed by loop excision or laser. However, where these have failed surgical excision is necessary and carries certain risks:

- general anaesthesia is necessary
- risk of haemorrhage and infection
- risk of damage to cervix (incompetent cervix)
- risk of cervical stenosis
- possible decrease in fertility (reduction in endocervical cells that produce cervical mucus, essential to the transport of sperm).

Hysterectomy (see p. 332) will sometimes be considered when:

- there are recurrent abnormal smears despite treatment, including cone biopsy
- the woman wants to be sterilized anyway
- there are associated gynaecological problems (e.g. fibroids, menorrhagia)
- there is suspicion of invasive disease.

Box 9.1 Information following treatment for CIN

- There may be a blood-stained discharge for a few days.
- Discharge after cryocautery is usually profuse and watery.
- Sexual intercourse should be avoided for at least 4 weeks.
- Tampons should not be used during the first period after treatment.
- Who to contact in the event of heavy bleeding.
- Follow-up details.

FOLLOW-UP

Follow-up is important for several reasons:

- to identify residual disease
- to identify new CIN
- to identify new invasive disease
- to reassure both the patient and the clinician (Austoker & Davey 1997).

The process may vary slightly according to local guidelines and policy:

- continuing cytology is essential
- colposcopy not routinely necessary
- continuing surveillance can be carried out in a primary care setting.

Suggested follow-up of local destructive therapy of CIN 2 or CIN 3:

1. Smear at 6 months.
2. If negative repeat smear at 12 months.
3. If negative repeat annually for at least 4 years.
4. If negative then routine recall (3 yearly).

Follow-up after hysterectomy for CIN 2 or CIN 3:

1. Vault smear at 6 months.
2. Vault smear at 12 months.
3. If negative discontinue all further vault smears.

Annual vault smears should be continued if there is any suspicion that the pre-malignant condition has not been completely removed (Austoker & Davey 1997).

Key points

- All grades of CIN are considered to be completely curable.
- Over 90% of women with CIN are satisfactorily treated at the first attempt (Luesley 1997.)

REFERENCES

Austoker J, Davey C 1997 Cervical smear results explained: a guide for primary care. Cancer Research Campaign, London

Chamberlain G (ed) 1995 Gynaecological tumours. In: Gynaecology by ten teachers, 16th edn. Arnold, London, Ch 6

Luesley D 1997 The abnormal cervical smear. In: Luesley D (ed) Common conditions in gynaecology. Chapman & Hall, London, Ch 9

NHSCSP 1996 Standards & quality in colposcopy. NHSCSP Publication No 2. NHSCSP Publications, Sheffield

Smith T 1997 Colposcopy. Nursing Standard 11 (45): 49–56

ULTRASOUND SCANNING

Ultrasound scanning is a procedure that has many uses in women's health. An electrical transducer is moved across the skin; through this ultrasound waves are deflected from organs inside the body and displayed as a picture on a computer screen. There is no radiation. The procedure is inexpensive, non-invasive and painless, and is highly accurate in distinguishing between cystic and solid masses. However, it does not distinguish between benign and malignant solid tumours. It can be carried out as an out-patient procedure.

Ultrasound can be used on breasts for:

- identification of cysts
- fine needle biopsy and aspiration may be carried out under ultrasound scan.

Ultrasound can be used on the pelvis:

- Ovaries:
  - identification of cysts and tumours
  - monitoring of follicular growth during ovarian stimulation with drugs
  - may have a role as part of screening for early detection of ovarian cancer
  - diagnosis of polycystic ovary syndrome (see p. 318).
- Uterus:
  - presence and shape of structure
  - presence of fibroids
  - thickness of endometrium
  - diagnosis of early pregnancy
  - retained products of conception.
- Pelvis:
  - presence and shape of structures (e.g. absent uterus in Turner's syndrome) (see p. 105)
  - abscesses.

Ultrasound scanning has an important role in the monitoring of normal pregnancy and in the identification of some fetal abnormalities.

Pelvic ultrasound can be performed in two ways (Chamberlain 1995):

- Transabdominal:
  - the woman needs to have a very full bladder so that the pelvic organs have been pushed slightly out of the pelvis
  - can be uncomfortable because of the full bladder ('full to bursting')
  - may be more appropriate – for the very young or very old
    - if there is a large mass in the pelvis
    - if vaginal scan is too difficult or unacceptable.
- Transvaginal:
  - probe is inserted into the vagina
  - greater proximity to the organs gives a much clearer image.

The procedure is usually carried out by:

- doctors
- specially trained nurses
- trained technicians.

Nursing issues

Spend some time thinking about the following:

- knowledge of the procedure (e.g. vaginal or pelvic scan)
- knowledge of any preparation necessary (e.g. full bladder)
- understanding the importance of preserving the woman's privacy and dignity during the procedure
- knowledge of how the woman will receive her results
- understanding of the anxiety and fear there may be about the results.

REFERENCE

Chamberlain G (ed) 1995 Gynaecology by ten teachers. Arnold, London, Ch 2

Index